TRUST ME
I'M NOT A DOCTOR

An Uncontrolled Study
of Modern Medicine

"Simplification is the ultimate sophistication"
Leonardo Da Vinci

TRUST ME
I'M NOT A DOCTOR

An Uncontrolled Study
of Modern Medicine

Tracey Northern

GREEN EYED PUBLISHING

LONDON 2023

CONTENTS

FOREWORDS

As a researcher, writer, film maker and author myself, Tracey has been an enormous influence and inspiration not only to my works, but also challenging me to question the validity of many of my core beliefs and consider how they manifest in my life and affect not only me ... but also the world around me.

We are not only the author and illustrator of children's books together but also friends, philosophers, co-voyagers of discovery and co-sceptics of the validity of the nature of this reality we are taught to accept as unwavering truth. That is the important core tenant and purpose of this book.

To Tracey, it is presented as the humble, modest musings of a philosopher with no agenda to sway the reader one way or another, but rather to question and perhaps sway her own former limiting belief structures, while letting the reader share the process of self-growth and conscious expansion in real time.

Make no mistake. These are not just mere musings. These 'scribblings', as she calls them, are incredibly well researched and deeply profound insights into subjects that most of us have not only taken for granted but never even considered that we should question the source of their cogency.

Tracey's writings have forced me to go back and correct errors in my own beliefs, assumptions and false claims in my own former films and writings and to move forward in future works with more understanding, more consciousness, more questioning.

While I'd love to brag that I had anything to do with this book, I cannot, although Tracey may tell you that some of my own works may possibly have inspired her to dig deeper into some of these subjects and check if she should be listening to me, or rather, should I be listening to her?

The beauty of her writing in this book is the selfless humility, opposite to the onslaught of preaching and propaganda pushed down our throats these days, Tracey isn't preaching to the reader. She is on a co-voyage of discovery with the reader and if a book could possibly ask you what you think without you being able to respond, her inviting writing style somehow gives you, the reader, a chance to do that ... at least in your head to yourself.

STEVE FALCONER – FILM MAKER – SPACEBUSTERS

I wish I could remember exactly when Tracey and I first connected, but it was definitely long before 'Covid'! It was probably about 10 years ago that we began exchanging comments in various anti-vaccination and HIV dissident FB groups.

What I do remember is that it was a great relief to find another voice out there in the wilderness who was talking about germs not being the cause of any disease.

Tracey's knowledge spans far more than just the 'germ theory' lie, she has deeply researched many topics, including animal abuse, a subject that is also close to my heart. As she explains in her Introduction, it has been a real disappointment that those who fight animal abuse have failed to appreciate the extent of the abuse that occurs within medical research laboratories.

Tracey and I began having Skype conversations soon after the Covid nonsense began to take hold and have spent many hours since March 2021 discussing various topics - nothing was off the table.

Tracey's directness and deep research has been a breath of fresh air within the dogma of fixed beliefs that many people espouse these days. She has helped me deepen and broaden my own views and allowed me to contemplate other perspectives. So I am truly grateful to her for the opportunities to re-examine my ideas and thoughts on topics, even if we sometimes hold slightly different opinions on some of them.

I must add that those differences have never challenged our friendship, which I greatly value. Sadly, the ability to remain friends despite differing views is becoming increasingly rare in the current climate of 'divide and conquer'.

Tracey writes from a personal viewpoint; she not only speaks to you, she also poses questions to inspire you to really contemplate the topics from a perspective you may not have previously contemplated.

Although her title invites you to 'trust her', she does not expect us to actually obey this directive; instead, her purpose is to show us that an unexamined trust in 'experts', especially those who have been indoctrinated into the medical establishment system, is almost invariably misplaced.

If you aren't already familiar with her work, you are in for a treat and maybe some surprises as she urges you to re-examine and even shed some of your old beliefs.

DAWN LESTER – CO. AUTHOR OF 'WHAT REALLY MAKES YOU ILL?'

TRUST ME I'M NOT A DOCTOR, An Uncontrolled Study of Modern Medicine is a humorous title for a serious critique and expose of modern medicine. Tracey has compiled her essays over the years and produced her uncontrolled study of modern medicine.

I have been questioning the existence of viruses for almost 20 years. Just as with Dawn Lester, it was indeed a relief and a pleasure to come across Tracey's work. It meant that there were other people out there, ordinary people with no medical qualifications, who were also questioning Modern Medicine and the Germ Theory.

The central dogma of Modern Medicine is the Germ Theory of Disease. Tracey explains why the Germ Theory is wrong, and that viruses do not exist. The Germ Theory is a more recent modification of the miasma theory of disease, which is that noxious air causes disease. The miasma theory held sway for thousands of years and its current form – the Germ Theory – was in its zenith during the covid era, as we all know too well.

The covid narrative is now collapsing. Tracey's book is written with her unique sense of humour. Tracey pokes fun at the experts and at the doctors, with chapters such as 'Ex-Spurts – Who Do You Listen To?'. Trust Me I'm Not A Doctor can be read in a few sittings and captivates you with its analysis. She does simplify a complex topic and demolishes the Germ Theory of Disease medical myth.

JAMES McCUMISKEY – AUTHOR OF 'THE ACHILLES' HEEL OF THE BIOMEDICAL PARADIGM & THE ULTIMATE CONSPIRACY - THE BIOMEDICAL PARADIGM'

Tracey Northern – Introduction

Never in a month of Sundays did I imagine I'd be writing a book, let alone a book like this. How on earth did that happen? It's a long story actually.

I've always been more philosophical than materialistic and I was once quite susceptible to fear-mongering. I grew up during the cold war years and believed we could all be blown to kingdom come at any moment at the whim of two presidents with their hands on the red button. I also had an instinctive fear of anyone in a white coat with a needle in their hand. I clearly remember kicking out with both legs at a nurse with a needle coming towards me with a 'booster'. She didn't get to stick me, not that day. I had a lot of empathy and at age 12 decided I did not want to eat animals, but my poor mother had no clue how to help me with that so it was carry-on-as-is or starve. I had to wait until I left home to become a vegetarian.

I got waylaid for a while by travelling around Europe, then off to America and 5 years later landed in London where I finally decided to do it, become a plant eater. I sought out others at the local health food shops and joined an organization called Animal Aid and learned about the horrific practise of vivisection. It became my life's mission to end it, somehow.

I came across a book by Hans Reusch called 'Slaughter Of The Innocents' and that was a major turning point. A chapter on vaccines was what really hit me and turned everything I thought I'd known on its head. Medical research was not only cruel, it was also all a lie. From then on I looked at everything with new eyes, the rose tinted specs were off and I saw clearly.

I became active in animal rights while mothering my two children and trying to protect them from the cruel, lying world I'd discovered. I wasn't ready for the sudden onslaught of bullying at my first 'well baby' visit though and under duress from 3 burly nurses I watched as they dropped a 'diphtheria vaccine' into my baby's mouth while I flat out refused any jabs. I didn't even know what diphtheria was. Only that I was threatened with a dead baby if I didn't give him the magic vaccine. I went into that place with a healthy baby boy but came out with a very sick one. That was when my research began in earnest. I eventually put 2 and 2 together and linked his illness to that one episode as fact, although my gut had always told me to never let it happen again.

When my second baby arrived she was never taken to the so-called 'well baby' visits and I was struck off the doctor's register for refusing to let them see her.

It was hard to find any information in the days before the internet but as soon as that was born I was on it, searching for answers while working my way up the animal activist ladder too. I joined Myspace and interacted with other people trying to change the world but became despondent at Animal Rights' refusal to address medical research and only concentrating on the testing of household and beauty products. It was as if medical research was the holy grail that must not be touched. I found I had to convince everyone of the uselessness of vivisection as well as the cruelty, but I needed more knowledge.

I've delved deep into vaccines and cancer research for years, learning all the 'science', annoying my fellow researchers with my endless questions until I finally understood why it didn't make sense. Because it was never based on anything solid. It was all a lie. It's not meant to make sense because it's NONsense.

Up until this point I'd just been chatting and arguing, mostly with pro-vaxxers, and then Facebook arrived. There came a point where I needed to get things down in writing for the sake of my own memory and to save time with over-long comments, so my first 'article' was born – a post on Facebook titled 'Modern Medicine is Not a Science; It is a Religion' (the first chapter of this book).

Over the next few years I started writing down what I had learned but hadn't written about all of my cancer knowledge until Sallie O'Elkordy asked me to go on her show to talk about it. I didn't think I could talk for a full hour without facts at my fingertips so I wrote down a lot of what I wanted to say. Much later those notes became another article 'What if Cancer is Not a Disease But a Cure?' and the start of a string of shows with 'Crazz Files' which spawned my most popular article, 'Germ Theory an Idiots Guide'

This led to my most prolific writing/scribbling era during the covid lockdowns and the ultimate discovery to end the whole modern medicine saga and all its trappings. In 2019, because of growing censorship, I had to move my 'notes' from Facebook to an online blog, Northern Tracey's Scribblings, on WordPress.

Now it's time to put it all into some cohesive order and make it into a book. I hope it will illustrate my own journey of understanding and help you to understand too, because with knowledge everything becomes so much simpler and most importantly you will find there is actually nothing to fear out there at all (except maybe fear itself).

TRUST ME I'M NOT A DOCTOR

MODERN MEDICINE IS NOT A SCIENCE; IT IS A RELIGION

All through history new ideas in medicine have been met with disbelief and horror. People working in the field who discover new ideas that threaten the dogma are treated with scorn at least and outright violence at worst.

Take Semmelweis as a classic example. He worked in a hospital where many women were dying in childbirth. After much thought and some research he decided something was linked between the cadavers and the mothers, namely people were working on both, switching from one to the other. He introduced (shock/horror) HANDWASHING. In other words, basic hygiene before insertion into the body. Death rates plummeted but nevertheless he was kicked out and even then hounded to insanity and death in an asylum. He is now considered the pioneer of asepsis in obstetrics. Poor sod.

Then there is Béchamp, a better qualified contemporary of Pasteur who simply disappears from history even though his theories were far superior and better thought out. Lauded in his day and deleted from the future.

It goes right back to the inquisition when herbalists and other natural healers were deemed to be working with the devil, tortured and murdered horribly. Not much has changed to this day. When any new ideas come along which threaten the status quo and dogma in modern medicine (allopathy) they are shot down, sometimes literally!! Up to today and in the last year, roughly 50 holistic practitioners have died and disappeared under mysterious circumstances. [1]

Doctors today are not taught to think, just to do, hence we have been thrown back into the dark ages when the church ran the medical system. Andrew Wakefield, although never ever saying he was anti-vaccine but to this day is still treated like a pariah, was struck off for discovering a link between Autism and bowel damage presented to him by parents who mentioned a vaccine. His crime? Daring to think.

---

[1] 50 Holistic Doctors Have Died In The Last Year, But What's Being Done About It?

www.anonhq.com/50-holistic-doctors-mysteriously-died-last-year-whats-done/

In Germany a working doctor of allopathy (Dr. Hamer) discovered new evidence of how disease occurs and the link to the brain. His research was all done empirically (scientifically and on humans not animals or test tubes). His discovery threatens the very basis of allopathic medicine, namely the germ theory and the theory of contagion. He has been kicked out, just as others were, and even imprisoned but his work is so important that it must not be ignored. German New Medicine is now in the midst of the same Pasteur/Béchamp debacle whereby people are publishing bastardised versions of the GNM theory with Hamer trapped in purgatory, unable to do much besides sue for copyright and watch as the charlatans fail to heal, thus discrediting his work.

Suppression of any new idea is ominous; it means modern medicine is a religion and a dogma and not a science at all. It is in fact a fraud and must be exposed. Dr. Stefan Lanka, trained in micro biology and virology, is trying to do just that along with another award winning virologist Dr Deusberg and investigative journalist Jon Rappaport amongst others. [2]

Fear is allopathy's only weapon, fear of germs/viruses and fear of death from disease symptoms allegedly caused by them. Although this is their biggest weapon, the monster has no teeth.

The germ theory has never been scientifically proven to this day. It was based on hypothesis before the tiny things could be seen but when the hypothesis did not hold up (as in the case of tuberculosis) they simply transferred the blame to an even smaller entity which still could not be seen, the virus.

The father of microbiology, Koch, set rules for proving bacteria etc. cause disease. They are called Koch's Postulates and they are very simple and still hold today yet they are not adhered to as they have always defeated any attempt to prove contagion. Still today they have not been able to isolate these tiny bogeymen viruses nor prove they cause any disease using their own scientific law.

Koch's Postulates (thus was vivisection born):

1. The organism must be regularly associated with the disease and its characteristic lesions.
2. The organism must be isolated from the diseased host and grown in culture.

---

[2] There Is No Evidence That The Medically Relevant (Vaccine) Viruses Even Exist. www.exoplitics.blogs.com

3. The disease must be reproduced when a pure culture of the organism is introduced into a healthy, susceptible host.

4. The same organism must be re-isolated from the experimentally infected host.

As these simple rules defeated the germ theory so absolutely, instead of rethinking the theory Fredricks and Relman just rewrote, or rather circumnavigated and annihilated the laws and worked around the obvious farce. So virology was born. If you want to read these farcical new *laws/guidelines* you are welcome to fry your brain on them. [3]

This cover-up, which most people have never heard of, could be the unveiling of the greatest scam committed on human society in all our history. Rockefeller, who built the enormous empire of the allopathic medical system we know today and its ugly sister the pharmaceutical business, is doing all in his power to hush this up and ban anything which is not patentable through all his channels of politics, education, internet and media.

It's up to us to learn about it, talk about it and start healing ourselves. Taking the power from the monster is easy, just stop feeding it by using their poisonous products or running crying to them every time you get a sniffle or a fever. Learn about how we really get sick from Béchamp. His work is being revived and spread across the internet.

Learn how to help the body through the healing process and not fear the symptoms by signing up to Jayne Donegan's excellent articles and join or start your own local Arnica group.[4]

Learn as much as you can while you still can.

---

[3] Koch's Postulates in the 21st Century
www.virology.ws/2010/01/22/kochs-postulates-in-the-21st-century/
[4] www.informedparent.co.uk & arnica.org.uk

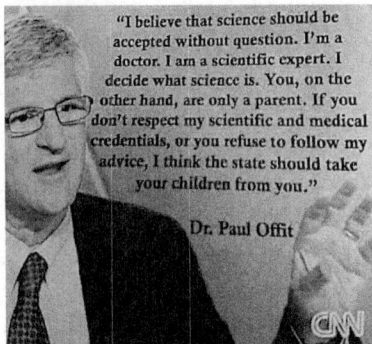

"I believe that science should be accepted without question. I'm a doctor. I am a scientific expert. I decide what science is. You, on the other hand, are only a parent. If you don't respect my scientific and medical credentials, or you refuse to follow my advice, I think the state should take your children from you."

Dr. Paul Offit

"When the medicine is so bad that they have to literally force it on us with new laws and powers you know it is time to do something. It is already too late! Despite the tendency of doctors to call modern medicine an 'inexact science', it is more accurate to say there is practically no science in modern medicine at all. Almost everything doctors do is based on a conjecture, a guess, a clinical impression, a whim, a hope, a wish, an opinion or a belief. In short, everything they do is based on anything but solid scientific evidence. Thus, medicine is not a science at all, but a belief system. Beliefs are held by every religion, including the Religion of Modern Medicine."

– Robert Mendelsohn MD preface by Hans Ruesch to 1000 Doctors (and many more) Against Vivisection.

P.S. The Science Delusion – Rupert Sheldrake's banned TedTalk on YouTube. A great talk about dogma in science. If only all scientists were like this.

"There is no such thing as consensus science.
If it's consensus, it isn't science.
If it's science, it isn't consensus. Period."
– Michael Crichton

THE SPANISH FLU (A BLUEPRINT FOR 2020?)

We've all now heard of the 'Spanish Flu' but why is it so popular right now especially with the 'producers' (Gates) and players in their 2020 theatrical masterpiece, Covid-19?

Let's see...

The Spanish Flu pandemic of 1918 actually originated at Fort Riley, Kansas where soldiers reported to the Army's largest training facility during World War I. The soldiers who were (DELIBERATELY) infected with the H1N1 influenza virus then served as countless vectors of dissemination for the pandemic that ultimately killed as many as 100 million people worldwide. That single US-executed biowarfare operation against humanity was arguably the deadliest depopulation event in human history. [5]

We've oft heard from some 'truthers' that the plandemic of 2020 was a bio-weapon attack but the lack of proof of an actual virus (as in the H1N1 above or the SarsCov2 today) or of its transmission makes it highly doubtful.

Also, if these scientists could come up with the bio-weapon they would also presumably hold the antidote. It would increase belief in their know-how and they would be holding all the cards which is what they need us to believe.

I do not believe they are capable of either. The obvious answer is it was simply poisonous chemicals injected using the smokescreen of 'vaccines'.

The 'vectors' mentioned above would be referring to vaccine 'shedding' (an admitted by-product mentioned in some inserts) and not a contagious viral transmission.

Chemical poisons have been known to pass from one close contact to another for years hence the need for hygiene in some workplaces.

"Eating should not be permitted in the smelters and as additional general precautionary measures the help should be

---

[5] 'Was the 2020 Wuhan Coronavirus an Engineered Biological Attack on China by America for Geopolitical Advantage?', presented by the alternative news outlet The Unz Review, Metallicman, 27 January 2020, citing article titled 'Spanish Flu of 1918 Was Really a Bioterror Attack on Humanity', presented by the Algora Blog, 6 February 2020.

required to wash the hands and to take a bath daily before leaving the smelter. It is also important that the help wear clothing made of close-meshed fabrics for the purpose of preventing the penetration of the underwear with soot and mercurial vapors. Where this precaution is not taken the workmen are apt to carry mercury into the home. In doing this the workman jeopardizes not only his own health by being continuously in an environment of mercury, but also that of the other occupants of the same house. At Idria cases of poisoning are often noted among members of a mercury worker's family. This is especially true where children sleep in the same bed with a father who is engaged in a mercury works. From what has been said it is evident that the untoward effects of mercury can be minimized if effective technical and hygienic appliances are installed in the smelter. It is also obvious that a complete prevention of disease from this cause is impossible."

– From the 1916 book 'Diseases of Occupation and Vocational Hygiene' by George Kober and William Hanson.

They had proof that poisoning can be passed from one person to another without any supposed invisible virus. It should also be noted that mercury was and still is an ingredient in vaccines whatever new fancy name they like to stick it under.

In the book 'Vaccination Condemned' by Eleanor McBean, PhD, N.D. the author describes, in detail, personal and family experiences during the 1918 'Spanish Flu' pandemic. McBean's coverage of the 1918 'Spanish Flu', as a reporter and an unvaccinated survivor, requires that the historical basis of the event needs to be revisited, not as a '*conspiracy theory*' but with evidence that will 'set your hair on fire'.

A few years ago, I came across another book by Eleanor McBean, 'Vaccination…The Silent Killer'. McBean provides evidence that not only were the historical events of the 1918 'Spanish Flu' compromised, but also those of the polio and swine flu epidemics. [6]

In preparation for WW1, a massive military vaccination experiment involving numerous prior developed vaccines took place in Fort Riley, Kansas – where the first 'Spanish Flu' case was reported. [7]

"There are still many unanswered questions on the causes of the 1918 Spanish Flu epidemic, and on the role of viruses in post-WWII polio (DDT neurotoxicity?).

---

[6] www.whale.to/a/mcbean2.html

[7] www.ncbi.nlm.nih.gov/pmc/articles/PMC2126288/pdf/449.pdf

These modern epidemics should have opened our minds to more critical analyses. Pasteur and Koch had constructed an understanding of infection applicable to several bacterial diseases. But this was before the first viruses were actually discovered. Transposing the principles of bacterial infections to viruses was, of course, very tempting but should not have been done without giving parallel attention to the innumerable risk factors in our toxic environment; to the toxicity of many drugs, and to some nutritional deficiencies. Cancer research had similar problems."

According to traditional conceptions, an infectious disease begins in one place and spreads out from there, depending on the environmental conditions, in certain directions. Such a development didn't occur with the Spanish Flu.

"In 1918, there were two different disease waves: a lighter one in spring and a much more severe wave, which claimed many lives, in late summer and autumn. Here, experts can't even agree whether the disease was introduced to the United States from Europe, or the other way around. According to one source, the epidemic began in February 1918 in the Spanish town of San Sebastian, close to the French border on the Atlantic coast. But another source names the same outbreak date, but a completely different place thousands of kilometers away from San Sebastian, on the other side of the Atlantic – New York City. That these outbreaks happened at the same time cannot be explained by either ship route or migrating bird patterns. Then in March 1918, there were reports of cases in two army camps in Kansas, hundreds of kilometers away from New York. In April, the Spanish Flu appeared in Paris for the first time, in May in Madrid, until it reached its peak in Spain at the end of May. In June, cases first began accumulating in war-torn Germany, but simultaneously in China, Japan, England and Norway as well. On 1 July, Leipzig had its first case. And over the course of that month, approximately half a million Germans were affected." [8]

The fledgling pharmaceutical industry, sponsored by the 'Rockefeller Institute for Medical Research' had something they never had before – a large supply of human test subjects. Supplied by the U.S. military's first draft, the test pool of subjects ballooned to over 6 million men. Between January 21st and June 4th of 1918, **Dr. Gates** (coincidence or a relative?) reports on an experiment where soldiers were given 3 doses of a bacterial meningitis vaccine. Those conducting the experiment on the soldiers were just spit-balling dosages of a

---

[8] Torsten Engelbrecht, German journalist/author; Claus Köhnlein, M.D, German physician/internist/author 'Virus Mania'

vaccine serum made in horses.

The vaccination regime was designed to be 3 doses.

4,792 men received the 1st dose, but only 4,257 got the 2nd dose (down 11%), and only 3702 received all three doses (down 22.7%).

A total of 1,090 men were not there for the 3rd dose.

What happened to these soldiers? Were they shipped East by train from Kansas to board a ship to Europe? Were they in the Fort Riley hospital?. **Dr. Gates** report doesn't tell us. [9]

"Autopsies after the war proved that the 1918 flu was NOT a 'FLU' at all. It was caused by random dosages of an experimental 'bacterial meningitis vaccine', which to this day, mimics flu-like symptoms. The massive, multiple assaults with additional vaccines on the unprepared immune systems of soldiers and civilians created a 'killing field'. Those that were not vaccinated were not affected." [10]

From January 21–June 4, 1918, an experimental bacterial meningitis vaccine cultured in horses by the Rockefeller Institute for Medical Research in New York was injected into soldiers at Fort Riley. They had around 6 MILLION soldiers to experiment on. WW1 U.S. soldiers were given 14-25 untested, experimental vaccines within days of each other, which triggered intensified cases of ALL the diseases at once.

They decided to reclassify this as a new disease (Spanish Flu). [11]

The catastrophe presented a very personal catastrophe for physicians.

"The pandemic, one of the worst to ever afflict the earth, was simply virtually erased from newspapers, magazines, books and society's collective memory" says Gina Kolata in her book 'Flu - The Great Influenza Pandemic of 1918 and the Search for the Virus that Caused It'.

This could be psychologically explained in two ways. The catastrophe presented a very personal catastrophe for physicians, because, although they were basically given all the money and material resources in their world to fight the alleged flu, they were unsuccessful in preventing the disaster. In a brutally clear way, doctors and

---

[9] www.ncbi.nlm.nih.gov/pmc/articles/PMC2126288/pdf/449.pdf

[10] www.salmartingano.com/2020/05/the-1918-spanish-flu-only-the-vaccinated-died/

[11] www.newscientist.com/article/dn14458-bacteria-were-the-real-killers-in-1918-flu-pandemic/

pharmacologists were shown the limits of their power. It is clear that mainstream medicine prefers not to dwell on such a total defeat, let alone expand upon it in memoirs or newspapers.

Restoring Faith in WHO?

Today we have dancing nurses, whistle blower doctors and scientists with a supposed chip on their shoulder. I wonder sometimes if this whole thing is a kind of reality advertising campaign for modern medicine which, let's face it, has been having an uphill battle with 'alternatives' as more and more people lose faith. Then this woman spurted out these words in 'Plandemic the Movie'…

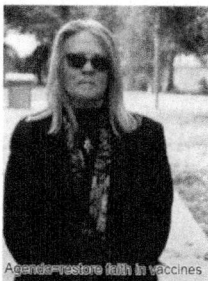

"We started an education company-we wake up doctors to restore faith in the promise of medicine"

Agenda-restore faith in vaccines

"I am not anti-vaccine, vaccines are immune therapy. My job is to develop immune therapies, that's what vaccines are."

The woman is Judy Mikovits and she worked alongside Dr. Fauci in the 1980's on the HIV/AIDS pandemic that never was. She makes out she is a whistle-blower but she has never blown the whistle on the fact that they never did find that elusive human immunodeficiency virus, yes HIV. She is only 'whistle-blowing' very selectively and the two quotes above were taken directly from her own film made for 'Truther TV' this year. Why would she want to 'restore faith' in medicine? If she is their poster child I'd wonder at the thoughts of their advertising agency and what cool-aid they were drinking. Listening to her rattle on is akin to your worst chemistry teacher scratching the blackboard.

In 1997, a paper by Jeffery Taubenberger's research team appeared in 'Science', claiming to have isolated an influenza virus (H1N1) from a victim of the 1918 pandemic.

"But before one can be certain that a pandemic virus had in fact been detected, some important questions must be asked," writes Canadian biologist David Crowe, who analyzed the paper.

The researchers had taken genetic material from the preserved lung tissue of a victim, a soldier, who died in 1918. Lung diseases were extremely typical of the Spanish Flu, but it is a big leap to conclude that the many other million victims also died from the same cause. And particularly 'the same virus' as Crowe points out.

In 1918 they also carried out numerous experiments to prove the flu was being transmitted person to person. Look at Milton J. Rosenau MD and Boston Medical Association's 1919 experimental study on the Spanish Flu not being a transmittable virus by prolonged physical contact, casual contact or even injection of infected fluids from the sick to healthy...

"The experiment began with 100 volunteers from the Navy who had no history of influenza. Rosenau was the first to report on the experiments conducted at Gallops Island in November and December 1918. His first volunteers received first one strain and then several strains of Pfeiffer bacillus by spray and swab into their noses and throats and then into their eyes.

When that procedure failed to produce disease, others were inoculated with mixtures of other organisms isolated from the throats and noses of influenza patients. Next, some volunteers received injections of blood from influenza patients.

Finally, 13 of the volunteers were taken into an influenza ward and exposed to 10 influenza patients each. Each volunteer was to shake hands with each patient, to talk with him at close range, and to permit him to cough directly into his face.

None of the volunteers in these experiments developed influenza. Rosenau was clearly puzzled, and he cautioned against drawing conclusions from negative results. He ended his article in JAMA with a telling acknowledgement: "We entered the outbreak with a notion that we knew the cause of the disease, and were quite sure we knew how it was transmitted from person to person. Perhaps, if we have learned anything, it is that we are not quite sure what we know about the disease." [12]

So the contagion experiments were already done and dusted back then, some more have been done lately but they are kept very quiet as the outcome is never satisfactory to the disease mongering medicine men who need us to trust in their expertise and do as we are told, despite any suspicions that all might not be as it seems.

---

[12] Diseases of the Respiratory System: Entry 1377. Experiments to Determine the Mode of Spread of Influenza. Milton J. Rosenau. J., in Abstracts of Bacteriology, Vol. III, Baltimore: Williams & Wilkins Company, 1919, p. 234.

What better way to make us run in fear to saviors in white coats than to tell us an invisible 'virus'/bogeyman is out to get us?

When I started looking into the Spanish Flu about five years ago or more I could only find ONE YouTube video giving this information. I went back to it often for reference but within a year it was deleted along with its maker a Swedish (?) man called Sacha (?).

The info is now getting out there again and it is much needed because someone is using the Spanish Flu 'episode' as a blueprint and we all know Bill Gates has a deep fascination for it, but does he know the truth about it or is he another useful idiot who believes in contagion?

Simply follow the money.

One doctor witnessing the events is quoted:

"If what is happening here is ever to become public, the history of vaccination would be over. Nobody will ever want to vaccinate again."

What is this quote referring to?

1917-18 in the Philippines, where the US pharma industry was conducting their vaccine experiments. They did their first mass vaccination test there killing ¾ of the population. The vaccines were not blamed as usual and the deaths attributed to a 'flu epidemic'. The same vaccines were then issued to the soldiers of WW1 and the deaths went on spreading from there.

SOMETHING YOU SHOULD KNOW

It came to my attention while researching for a possible podcast that the whole Convid fiasco almost certainly started as a cover-up of the first public trial of China's, and the worlds, first SARS/Cov vaccine (or was it a cover-up of something else, or both?). They have been working on a 'coronavirus' vaccine ever since the first SARS 'outbreak'. An article on investmentwatchblog.com found me somehow and I wondered how it had been sitting there for so long with no interest. It certainly sparked mine. [13]

It's funny how some of the financial papers are where you can find the real info. In them they claim: **"According to the Law, China is to implement a state immunization program and <u>residents living within the territory of China are legally obligated to be vaccinated with immunization program vaccines which are provided by the government free of charge</u>."**

Sadly they miss the ball on how this affects people, only claiming it makes them more susceptible to other coronaviruses. This would not explain how so many became ill all at the same time and as we already know no virus has ever been purified and proved to CAUSE any illness.

In this article the actual law has a section which is very interesting because it mentions a kind of 'track and trace' technology IN the vaccine. Was this the test run for the so-called 'vaccines' now being foisted on us and the cause of the original deaths in Wuhan which sparked this whole plandemic?

"The Law mandates the launching of a national vaccine electronic tracking platform that integrates tracking information throughout the whole process of vaccine production, distribution and use to ensure all vaccine products can be tracked and verified." [14]

This is the famous Chinese study which everyone refers to as the one in which all the animals died. [15]

They claim they died when they were 'challenged with the wild virus'. Most people assume that this means they were exposed to a virus

---

[13] www.investmentwatchblog.com/chinas-mandatory-vaccination-law-went-into-effect-on-december-1-2019-the-coronavirus-outbreak-is-a-vaccine-experiment-gone-bad/

[14] www.loc.gov/law/foreign-news/article/china-vaccine-law-passed/

[15] www.pubmed.ncbi.nlm.nih.gov/22536382/

in the air or similar as they assume we are all supposedly challenged by a 'wild virus'. This is however far from what really happens. They have no 'wild virus' to start with and all and every experiment to try and induce disease in humans or animals by using the mucus and even excrement of sick people, even by injection, has failed miserably. Why would they therefore do that? No, what they actually do is vaccinate them again with the same vaccine (including all its chemicals and proteins).

In the study they claim the original vaccination caused 'immunopathological' changes.

It's strange that they don't seem to know about Richet's paper on anaphylaxis back in 1913 which won a Nobel prize and coined the term 'allergy', in which he shows an injection of anything can cause the body to over-react if injected a second time. You all know what anaphylaxis is but did you know it never existed before vaccines? Neither did allergies to foods.

The conclusion to that study warns of caution to move to human studies: **"These SARS-Cov vaccines all induced antibody and protection against infection with SARS-Cov. However, challenge of mice given any of the vaccines led to occurrence of Th2-type immunopathology suggesting hypersensitivity to SARS-Cov components was induced. Caution in proceeding to application of a SARS-Cov vaccine in humans is indicated."**

Read Charles Richet's Nobel lecture on Anaphylaxis from December 11th 1913. [16]

It's important to understand that every person who studies medicine should know this and also therefore know how vaccines prime us to be killed by something as harmless as a peanut. Peanut oil was an unnamed ingredient in some vaccines. They did not have to declare it as it was GRAS (generally regarded as safe).

The Chinese were working on several SARS/Cov vaccines and have lodged 3 SARS/Cov genetic sequences with the online gene bank. They are named SARS/Cov1, 2 and 3. All the genetic sequences were manufactured using CRISPR which means they take bits of genes from animals and humans and splice them together. This is where the silly conspiracy comes from that covid is a bio-weapon made in a Chinese lab, and where the bat legend came from as, yes, there are some bat sequences in there, HOWEVER a gene sequence is NOT A VIRUS.

---

[16] www.nobelprize.org/prizes/medicine/1913/richet/lecture/

That is where the bio-weapon theory falls down.

It is ridiculous.

The fact that we are being told the vaccines for covid were rushed through is a lie. They've been working on them for almost 20 years (with no success).

The fact that we are being told SARS/Cov2 is a 'novel virus' is also a lie. The SARS/Cov2 gene sequence has been available to gene labs since 2007 at least and these gene sequences are being passed off as 'viruses'. That is why the PCR is not a test for disease, it is a lab tool for finding certain gene sequences and NOT VIRUSES.

The next area to declare an outbreak after Wuhan was Bergamo in Italy. An Italian doctor confirmed that there had been a vaccine drive there too, shortly before people started getting very ill. It was a drive of two vaccines, one for meningitis and another for pneumonia and was given to the very old and sick who were exactly the people who allegedly started dying from 'covid'.

Both Wuhan and Bergamo are also very highly polluted AND both areas were trialing 5G. Now we have to wonder which of these three things were they trying to cover-up? 5G was being tested at many hospitals, particularly those using ambulances, so many built up areas, major cities and hospitals around the world were becoming affected, but by what? Any of these three factors could be causing breathing problems and a combination of all three would obviously be worse.

If you look at the pictures in the vaccine paper of the poor mice lungs they look eerily similar to the ones they were claiming were covid lungs in New York. In 2019 New York was pushing vaccine mandates and even removed religious exemptions. [17]

Then in the UK and USA the flu jab was 'upgraded' for the 2019 season with larger doses of 'adjuvants' (gene sequences made in a lab which are supposed to replicate a 'virus'). This would be akin to multiple foreign proteins being injected priming for anaphylaxis.

This was recommended in Autumn 2019 for everyone over 65 and never tested; it could have been the cause of even more deaths than the usual flu shots cause. [18]

---

[17] www.npr.org/2019/04/19/715016284/brooklyn-judge-upholds-mandatory-vaccinations-as-new-york-city-closes-more-schoo?t=1611502070220

[18] www.aarp.org/health/conditions-treatments/info-2020/high-dose-flu-vaccines.html

Every care home worker knows that frail old residents start dying en masse straight after the jabs.

Back to my original point.

Was this a cover-up for a vaccine trial gone wrong or was it a cover-up of effects of 5G trials? Or both? At what point did they decide this was the pandemic to 'go-live' with their Great Reset? How long have they been working on the RNA gene therapy shot which they are telling us is a vaccine when it is nothing of the sort? Why two shots when they know that can and will cause anaphylaxis?

Does this article open any eyes or does it just pose more questions than it answers?

The Germ Theory – An Idiots Guide

How did we get ourselves into this pickle we're in? What is the main ingredient, the heart that is pumping the fear around the world right now? IT IS The Germ theory. Without this they would never have been able to build up the fear to the hysterical level it has reached.

They would never have been able to build the all-encompassing and powerful big pHarma and they would never have had so much power to wield over the entire earth. THIS is why it is so important that we understand what germ theory is and what it is not.

What is the germ theory of disease? The Britannica definition says: **"Germ theory, the theory that certain diseases are caused by the invasion of the body by microorganisms, organisms too small to be seen except through a microscope."**

Merriam Websters dictionary definition **"a theory in medicine: infections, contagious diseases and various other conditions result from the action of microorganisms"**

One thing the medical establishment always throws at us is their favourite quote "Correlation does not equal causation" which means basically just because something is there does not mean it is the cause.

They use this to poo-poo any claims that their drugs might be making us sick yet totally ignore it when it comes to germ theory. In fact germ theory only works if you break that rule and blame the first thing you see. Just like the old analogy of blaming the firemen for the fire they come to put out or blaming the flies for the garbage.

Some people might be surprised to know germ theory and all that's been built on is less than 150 years old OFFICIALLY and just like the information war going on today, with censorship, the story of how germ theory gained so much ground is also heavily censored. No-one in medical school or even any school is ever taught about a scientist called Béchamp who in his day was more important than Einstein. He was infinitely cleverer and years ahead of the man who everyone does talk about – Pasteur.

Pasteur was a fame and power hungry showman with a big mouth and a bad temper. He was also extremely cruel to the point even his contemporaries complained after his sawing the skulls off live dogs and even using condemned prisoners for vivisecting.

He was not well liked and certainly not a great scientist so how did he and this theory get so famous? There is no written proof of it but all the signs point to outside influence and help, strings were pulled and connections made. He was either introduced into the 'club' or was one of their puppets used for his showmanship to usher in their control mechanism which was to be THE GERM THEORY, the bogeyman, the invisible enemy, the perfect weapon as well as a scapegoat for all the growing industries which were truly hurting people (THEIR industries).

It is well known that the Rothschilds were strongly linked with European Royalty and Napoleon at the time, influencing everything from wars to education, so no doubt they had a hand in the rise of Pasteur and his germ theory which also explains the quick take up of the cause in America by the Rockefellers and other countries where the families held power.

Anything you read about Pasteur's experiments, which were put on like large shows to crowds of people, is either fake news or censored. Like his anthrax experiments on sheep. We are told they were a raging success and his anthrax vaccine did make him a large fortune.

A few years ago though, in 1971, his journals which had been passed down with the condition that they were to be kept secret, were in fact made public as the last male heir died. Those journals were a bombshell to the germ theory. They exposed the way he cheated, lied and plagiarized fellow scientists, especially Béchamp.

Remember those sheep? In his first experiment he vaccinated 4,564 sheep of which 3,696 dropped dead almost instantly. He had to pay for all the sheep he'd killed so for his next public experiment he simply cheated.

So basically Pasteur was the original poster child for a marketing campaign for the pharmaceutical companies ultimate brainchild. The vaccine. The foundation was set. Vaccines were to be the basis of the new health system based entirely on the unproven germ theory.

So what about this Béchamp fella and why was he so ignored?

Well because his work was proving the complete opposite of what Pasteur was selling so hard. Germs were NOT the cause of disease. While Pasteur was busy hobnobbing with Napoleon, partying with his mates and doing his showcase experiments Béchamp was beavering away in his lab looking at these germs under the newly invented microscope.

He saw that the microbes were not in fact all different species. He saw them change from one form into another like caterpillars into butterflies, like seeds into plants except they didn't only change once or twice, they had MANY different forms. They seemed to start as a seed or a spore, the tiniest form which he called a microzyma. Then they went through a number of different shapes, a TB shape which is a rod shape, a Y shape which they now claim is an antibody and various other shapes Pasteur claimed to be different species, until a final form which bursts forth more of those spores, and so back to the beginning.

This is called PLEOMORPHISM. This one discovery should have put the germ theory to bed right there because how can they blame a specific species of a microbe as being a cause of a specific disease if it is not a specific species but just one face of the same microbe? It didn't kill the germ theory though because it was ignored, buried and censored and nowadays pleomorphism gets referred to as 'good and bad bacteria'.

Béchamp also discovered that the germs did not invade from outside but were already IN the body and produced IN and BY the body. He also showed that the morphing into different forms happened when the tissue they were in was dead or dying or if poisons were introduced. He observed them morphing and cleaning up dead tissues and cells and even neutralizing some poisons. The germs were not CAUSING anything, they were cleaning up the mess caused by something else. They are like the clean-up crew after a bomb blast and in some cases they have to don hazmat suits in order to get the job done. This is why they morph, to protect themselves from the hazards they are cleaning up and to survive hostile terrains.

Robert Koch came into the fray and his contribution was to set up scientific rules which would verify germ theory; these rules are called Koch's Postulates.

One big problem with that was that however hard they tried they could not even make the first rule stick. Looking at Tuberculin, the rod shaped bacteria they thought was causing TB, they could not find it in every person who showed the symptoms, and they also found it in perfectly healthy people. Now you see why after all this time it's still called a theory and not a law. It has never fulfilled any of the laws set up to prove it. This is why we get convoluted explanations to explain themselves out of this fact. It's called circular reasoning and the art of bullshitting.

Meantime across the pond in America, Rockefeller and his 'club' (no doubt under the direction of the Rothschilds) were quickly setting up their modern medical empire on the foundation of this germ theory which was being mirrored all over the countries the Rothschilds had power and influence in. Using philanthropy as their cover they were effectively buying up all the universities and closing down all the herbalist and homeopathic schools and hospitals (because they were far too successful at helping people get well very cheaply using NATURAL substances which could not be patented, and so controlled and profited from by the now powerful pharma companies which were also being bought up by Rockefeller, who had seen the opportunity to make new drugs from ingredients from his oil refining business).

Follow the money. You can read all about this process in detail in a book called The Medicine Racket and in the (now hard to find) film, Rockefeller Medicine.

Modern orthodox medicine IS a racket and was built using mafia tactics which are the workings behind philanthropy. Notice how much power Bill Gates's philanthropic donations has bought him today. Same process being used again to gain power and wealth.

During this time (early 1900's) there were also many experiments being carried out to find the actual mode of contagion in the germ theory, and how these diseases were being passed from one person to another.

They are all in the chapter 'Contagion – A Fairy Story', but here's a snippet of one of the experiments I've picked out because of the interesting conclusion they stumbled upon and it's quite relevant to our situation.

In 1930, Dochez et al. attempted to infect a group of men experimentally with the common cold. The authors stated in their results something that is nothing short of amazing. **"It was apparent very early that this individual was more or less unreliable and from the start it was possible to keep him in the dark regarding our procedure. He had inconspicuous symptoms after his test injection of sterile broth and no more striking results from the cold filtrate, until an assistant, on the second day after injection, inadvertently referred to this failure to contract a cold. That evening and night the subject reported severe symptomatology, including sneezing, cough, sore throat and stuffiness in the nose. The next morning he was told that he had been misinformed in regard to the nature of the filtrate and his symptoms subsided within the hour. It is important to note that there was an entire absence of objective pathological changes."**

In other words they couldn't see anything (untoward) going on under a microscope. It seemed in this case they had found people could be made sick by mere suggestion. Hmmm, interesting don't you think?

All the other experiments completely failed to make people sick unless they were injected or had it shoved right up their noses as in this experiment.

In 1920, Schmidt et al conducted two controlled experiments, exposing healthy people to the bodily fluids of sick people. Of 196 people exposed to the mucous secretions of sick people, 21 (10.7%) developed colds and three (1.5%) developed grippe (flu). In the second group, of the 84 healthy people exposed to mucous secretions of sick people, five developed grippe (5.9%) and four colds (4.7%). Of forty-three controls who had been inoculated with sterile physiological salt solutions eight (18.6%) developed colds. A higher percentage of people got sick after being exposed to saline compared to those being exposed to the 'virus'. (I wonder if the word virus is being used in the old sense or the new here).

So the placebo group were the worst affected! Of all the various experiments not one person became sick from personal contact even to the point of swapping spit.

Then there is the curious 1950's case of Masha and Dasha…

"The new mother was told that her twin babies had died after birth. However the truth was far different: they were sent to an institute near Moscow to be studied. This was to be the fate of Masha and Dasha, one of the most unusual sets of "Siamese" or conjoined twins ever born.

Identical twins are formed when a fertilized egg divides into two eggs. The two eggs grow into two babies that are identical in every respect. Conjoined or Siamese twins are formed in the same way as identical twins but the eggs, for some reason, don't completely separate; instead, they remain partially attached. It was the unique way in which the twins were connected that caused Soviet scientists to take such an interest in them.

Although Masha and Dasha have four arms, they have only three legs. They stand on two of their legs, one controlled by Masha, one by Dasha (they were five before they learned how to walk) while a third, vestigial leg remains in the air behind them. Their upper intestines are separated but they share a single lower intestine and rectum. They have four kidneys and one bladder, and often disagree on when to urinate. They have a common reproductive system.

Because their circulatory systems are interconnected, the twins share each other's blood. Therefore, a bacterium or virus

**that enters one twins' bloodstream will soon be seen in the blood
of her sister. Yet surprisingly, illness affects them differently.
Dasha is short-sighted, prone to colds and right-handed. Masha
smokes occasionally, has a healthier constitution, higher blood
pressure than her sister, good eyesight and is left-handed.**

**The twins differing health patterns present a mystery. Why did
one become ill with a childhood disease, like measles for
example, while the other did not? The measles 'bug' was in both
of their bodies, in their collective bloodstream; so why didn't both
get the measles? Evidently there is more to 'getting the measles'
than having the measles 'bug'. This phenomenon was seen over
and over again with the girls (flu, colds, other childhood diseases
were all experienced separately). If germs alone had the power to
cause infectious diseases, why would one of the twins be disease-
free while the other was ill?"** [19]

Royal Raymond Rife also came along in the 1930's and invented a
new microscope, which miraculously could see live microbes down to
much smaller sizes which could potentially blow their cover again. He
could see the tiniest microbes which we now know are the microzyma
(other scientists have given them names too – protits, somatids).

His life's work and his microscope were seized by the FBI, never to
be seen again. Poor Rife's reputation was destroyed, he was driven to
drink and he wasn't even anti-germ theory! He was however a threat to
the drugs business. Why did the medical industry not want to use this
amazing new technology but plumped for the electron microscope
instead which can only see dead tissues, nothing living and moving?

I think you know.

I'll just mention in passing that more recently Gaston Naessens has
also built a similar microscope and is actually videoing pleomorphism
and has even mapped out all the different forms they take, but that's
something you can look into yourself.

This exposing of the germ theory as false had to be nipped in the
bud so what did they do? They invented VIRUSES. They had to be
smaller than the wavelength of light so no-one could see them under a
normal microscope, so the INVISIBLE ENEMY was reborn and a
new business could also be built on it called VIROLOGY.

It was also in the 1930's coincidentally that the dictionary definition

---

[19] www.drmadalynperrydc.com/performance-health-library/the-
chiropractic-story-of-masha-and-dasha/

of VIRUS was changed by Rockefeller, Rivers and Flexner from the old definition of "A liquid poison" to this new one "Any of various submicroscopic agents that infect living organisms, often causing disease, and that consist of a single or double strand of RNA or DNA surrounded by a protein coat. Unable to replicate without a host cell, viruses are typically not considered living organisms."

Hmm not living? Then not a microbe and also what's all that nonsense about 'living viruses' and 'live virus' vaccines? More circular reasoning no doubt.

Virology is the ultimate pseudo-science. Built on the now crumbling foundations of germ theory and sellotaped together with the newly developed science of genetics, it is the business of chasing unicorns, things that do not exist and that no-one can refute without having journeyed into the belly of the beast and seen the cogs in the machine making the fantasy sci-fi production called The Virus Hunters (if it were a Hollywood production, which it kind of is).

Stefan Lanka did exactly that, he went backstage and saw all the actors without their make-up and he knew it was all a massive con trick. There are no viruses, there never were. They've even taken the pleomorphism which is starting to creep out of oblivion and slapped it onto their story about viruses.

"Why do their vaccines not work? Oh the virus has morphed/mutated" they like to say now, but it's the very thing which could have brought down the original germ theory and they have managed to prop up germ theory mark two with. It's like a magic trick but not a very good one. It's also a slap in the face to poor old Béchamp.

They are mocking us.

Everyone who is arguing over the details, like ingredients, safety and efficacy of different vaccines or drugs is either still ignorant or has one foot in and one foot out of this business. Especially when we know they have been shown the proof germ theory is a lie and viruses don't exist.

There are many out there who are controlling the narrative, hiding details from us still. These are called gatekeepers and controlled opposition. They are easy to spot once you know everything I've told you here is fact. Like those in the anti-vaccine movement who boldly shout that they are not anti-vax, that they want safer vaccines. That is controlled opposition. If they really wanted to end dangerous vaccines they would tell the truth that they never worked and never will, but hey that would be too easy and they would have to go and get a proper job.

There are those who harp on about bad bacteria and healthy microbiomes. There are no 'good and bad bacteria'. There are only bacteria in various forms affected by the environment they are in. This refers to Béchamp's Terrain Theory. Bacteria are just seen in varying forms like wearing protective gear. Even fungus is one of these forms and is the one needed for the most toxic clean ups. Just like fungus can be used to clean up giant oil spills in the sea or how fungi clear up the dead stuff on the forest floor where there is no light. When they speak of an 'infection' they are referring to a clean-up site where lots of bacteria are working hard to sort out some mess.

For example if you get a splinter in your finger and try as you might you just can't get it out, what happens? A blister will form, it will be sore because it is 'inflamed', that is the extra blood transporting things in and out of the site, a white bubble forms around the splinter, this is full of microbes breaking the splinter down, if it can't be broken down then the skin will grow under it and eventually the body pushes out the splinter. I have seen this happen on my own fingers. THIS is your so-called 'immune system'. There is no such thing as an immune system though, because there is nothing to be immune to and the things they call diseases CAN happen more than once.

The immune theory was built on the findings of the ability to become drug resistant. If you take a drug regularly in small doses your body becomes accustomed to it and to get the effect the drug produces you need to take more and more. Like you become immune to the effects of the poisons. This is the body learning how to deal with a specific toxin more efficiently and is a well-known process, they just tagged it onto the germ theory and applied it to germs, but as we know germs do not cause disease, it does not apply and you cannot be immune from being poisoned again. You do not 'strengthen your immune system' as the naturopaths like to say. You just stop poisoning yourself and you give your body good clean species appropriate food. What we have been taught is an 'immune system' is actually a garbage collection system and a hazardous waste disposal system.

If there is no immune system and we do not build up immunity to germs (our own clean-up crew) then vaccines are a complete and utter scam. Why do you think they have to put ADJUVANTS into vaccines to make the fictitious immune system react to the injection of some 'germs'? Adjuvants in English are toxic ingredients like heavy metals. One of them is the favourite of the orthodox quacks of old…mercury.

They actually gave it out like sweets back in the day for all manner of illness along with cocaine and heroin, three very popular medicines. No wonder everyone was scared of the quacks. By the way, the name Quack comes from the German for mercury which is Quackenselber. Funny how they now call naturopaths or anyone using a different method a quack. Just like the projecting or mirroring that those satanists use. Just saying.

They have been hiding mercury in vaccines for years. So when they give a vaccine, the body is not reacting to the germs it is reacting to a massive toxic explosion entering the body from a direction that is the most difficult to deal with, right into the tissues and the blood stream so bypassing our natural defense barriers (skin, mucous membranes, digestive system).

Pro-vaxxers like to say about this deadly poison in vaccines that "the poison is in the dose" basically meaning a tiny dose of poison is not necessarily poisonous. BUT it was proven, also in the early 1900's, that the mode of entry of poison can change all that. Look up Richet and his Nobel Prize winning talk on anaphylaxis. They have known since back then that injection of ANYTHING (especially proteins alarmingly) can induce the body to have a severe reaction if it encounters the same substance a second time.

Now thinking about how they give vaccines one after the other and that they are not injecting viruses but proteins (remember the description of a virus?). They also put common foodstuffs in there (like peanut oil), do you think that might cause some serious problems? AND how have they ignored this Nobel prize winning work? Odd isn't it? Do they know or not? It's obviously not in the script. Another inconvenient truth?

If you are listening to doctors or mainstream scientists for your info you are still watching the Muppet show directed and produced by Rockefeller medicine. They reel you in with their pretty CGI pictures, and qualifications and bamboozle you with fancy long Latin words and circular reasoning. They like to tell people like me and you dear reader that we are stupid because we are not qualified so can't possibly understand science. A nurse actually said this to me the other day.

These people have been thoroughly indoctrinated into the cult and don't know how to tell the truth without admitting their whole career has been a lie, that they have been killing people not healing them. They call doctors officially the 3rd leading cause of death. But they are only 3rd officially because they claim cancer and heart disease kill slightly more people. But there again those deaths were also from the treatments meted out by doctors and not their own bodies healing processes so medical doctors are in fact the number one cause of death today. That is a hard pill to swallow so you can see why they'd prefer not to go there. The only doctors and scientists worth listening to are the ones who retired or got out when they found out the truth. Even naturopaths and many so called alternative medicine doctors are steeped in germ theory and all its trappings.

The truth is ultimately our bodies are miraculous self-healing organisms. The body does not need help to heal except in extreme circumstances of injury which is life-threatening. In fact when you think you are sick or 'diseased' as you are having symptoms, those are the actual signs of the body healing itself and your microbiome doing its thing. Pushing out poisons through the skin is an obvious process we can see happening with things like chickenpox or indeed anything called a pox, even acne, is the same process of cleansing. Lots of different names for the same thing. ALL the symptoms we see which they call disease are in fact the body healing itself from something and guess who is doing all the work in there? Yes those 'germs'.

Those acute illnesses which they claim to be contagious diseases, if you notice, they are all explosions of toxins exiting the body, through the skin, the mouth, the lungs, the bowels just about every hole we have. When doctors interfere with their drugs, which stop all these processes, they are effectively closing all the exits and forcing the body to deal with it somehow in another way.

This is where chronic illness comes in. Those toxins have to be dealt with, somehow, so temporarily they CAN be stored in the fat which keeps them out of reach of the organs, if they are too toxic for that they can be cordoned off into what we know as tumours or cysts.

The body then has to deal with the new toxins which have been added to the mix by the administered drugs. It's a kind of prioritizing in the body, lock the first offenders up temporarily and go deal with the new assault. The drugs actually put the body in stress mode (fight or flight) which is why we seem to feel better when we take the drugs. We tend to feel energized when we are under stress. It hasn't however cured anything. The build-up of toxic load will have to be dealt with by the body sometime down the line (when the body comes out of stress mode, which is usually when we are on holiday) and the bigger the load the bigger and more dramatic the symptoms will be.

It is like an accident waiting to happen except it is no accident.

There is so much to learn about what we are only now being shown thanks to the internet and those pesky conspiracy nuts. It may seem overwhelming but it isn't because it is so much simpler than a convoluted theory propped up by circular reasoning and blatant lies. The truth is always simpler than lies. The truth has always been here, written and spoken about by people practicing what they call alternatives but that are really just the truth.

I'd especially recommend you look into Natural Hygiene which is not what you may think from the name. When you hear hygiene nowadays you automatically think of killing germs right? THAT is not what the word actually means. Look it up, be amazed to see how they've twisted things. It's no good looking to science for proof as that is all controlled within the system built on germ theory (and controlled by the 'club') unless you learn their language and how to read their studies and spot the gaping mistakes. That can take years of practice and study and needs confidence and conviction.

I'd like to end with a couple of **quotes from 'What Really Makes You Ill? Why Everything You Thought You Knew About Disease Is Wrong' by Dawn Lester and David Parker**, which sum things up nicely I think.

"It is a fundamental principle that the burden of proof lies with those who propose a theory, yet in the case of Germ Theory that proof does not exist, there is no original scientific evidence that definitively proves that any germ causes any specific disease. There are however many reasons for the germ theory to be perpetuated as IF it has been scientifically established and proven to be true, some of those reasons relate to economics, politics and geo-politics." [20]

It's all about the money and power.

I just want to open your eyes a little and hope you will go and look into what I've said here. It's so important to wrench ourselves out of this sick and twisted paradigm they have built all around us before it kills us all. I sometimes feel the tipping point is near. Other days I feel despair that we're never gonna get it. I also suspect they know the game is up and the cash cow is almost dead on its feet and this might just be the final death throes of the dying paradigm.

Or is it just their genocidal plan of depopulation finally playing out?

---

[20] www.whatreallymakesyouill.com

They have hinted all along that the health industry is to change. What that change brings though is up to us. We have to base it on truth, not profits. We have to also lose the fear and trust our own bodies. We are perfectly designed as is all nature. Germ theory is not natural, it doesn't follow any of the rules of nature. It is a man-made dogma within a cult. Mother Nature or God, if you believe in him, didn't make any mistakes, WE did.

Contagion

14 Reasons Why Millions Of People (Never) Died From Infectious Diseases

Someone posted this lovely little article and I found it full of great info except for the one glaring cognitive dissonance of firmly believing in germ theory and contagion. I could never share it as is so decided to dissect it myself. I'll leave the writing as it was and add my own remarks in brackets.

Why did so many people once die from diseases like smallpox? Were the people vaccine-deficient, or is there more to this story? A glimpse into history soon reveals why disease was so rampant during the 1800's, and early 1900's. In Victorian England, the average life expectancy of the working class was just 16 years old. Those who made it to 30 or 40 years of age were 'old' and worn out. Here's why:

OVERCROWDING

During the 19th century, the population of London swelled by more than eight-fold, from 800,000 to 7 million inhabitants. All across the western world, as the Industrial Revolution took hold, vast numbers of rural folk moved into towns and cities, on the promise of a better life. For many, it turned into a nightmare. With housing in short supply, unscrupulous landlords leased every spare inch to desperate families – dingy damp cellars, fire-trap attics and under-stair storage rooms, many without any ventilation or light. Can you imagine the mouldy, stale **(and polluted)** air that these people were constantly breathing – no wonder so many had lung problems!

LACK OF PLUMBING

Entire streets had to share one outdoor toilet, which was usually in foul condition – cleaning supplies were expensive, and flies hung around in droves (and then made their way through open windows to nearby kitchens etc)…and of course, there was always somebody with a bad case of diarrhoea. Sewerage drained into waterways via open channels in the streets and lanes, or simply lay stagnant in stinking cesspools of filth.

(I would add here that in older times pigs were kept to keep the streets clean of human waste. This is why in many cultures pigs are never eaten and considered 'unclean'. They were the original sewage workers).

CONTAMINATED DRINKING WATER

With no environmental laws in place, raw sewage poured into drinking water supplies, as did run-off and toxic waste from factories and animal slaughterhouses. **(One of the observations from the 'black death' was that people who lived in and close to the pubs did not succumb. Could this have been because they drank alcohol instead of dirty water?)**

CONTAMINATED FOOD SUPPLY

(Contaminated with what?). With slow, unreliable transport, and no refrigeration, food was often past its use-by date. **(In other words spoiled/rotten/decomposing).** Diseased **(not diseased just rotting)** and rotting meat was made into sausages and ham. Before pasteurization, milk was treated with formaldehyde to prevent souring. **(Wow, I did not know this one!!).** Fresh produce **(by which they mean living foods, fruit and vegetables)**, when it was available, was often slimy and not fit for human consumption. **(A friend of mine seemed to think that the milkmaids in the famous story did not get smallpox because they drank so much milk. That's a very blinkered theory. They lived in the countryside with plenty of fresh air and fresh food. Milk was not a cure for 'smallpox' which was simply poisoned skin from all the chemical pollution).**

ABSENT MOTHERS

Because doctors were offended at the suggestion that they had dirty hands, in need of washing, about 1 in 3 mothers died from infection after childbirth. **(Yes their hands were dirty with chemicals and poisons from working on cadavers down the hall. Nothing to do with germs).** Their infants had a 4x higher risk of dying, usually from infections **(no, from poisoning)**. If the baby survived past infancy, they could usually look forward to a life of malnutrition, hard labour and improper care, often performed by older siblings. During the Industrial Revolution, many mothers worked long hours in factories, leaving their young children in the care of hired 'nurse-girls', who were little more than children themselves, between 8-12 years of age.

CHILD LABOUR

With the Industrial Revolution in full swing and labour in

short supply, children as young as four and five were put to work in sweatshops and factories. Many of the jobs involved long hours, working in dangerous conditions, such as around heavy machinery or working near furnaces. Children were regularly crushed to death, or had limbs severed, in some of the more dangerous industries, such as underground mining. Basically, millions of children had no childhood, but a monotonous, depressing existence. **(Also as illustrated in the book Diseases of Occupation and Vocational Hygiene workers in 'dirty' jobs could bring that pollution home and pollute their family).**

POLLUTED AIR

Factories spewed soot and waste into the air, unchecked and unregulated. Cities were covered in a layer of grease and grime. Lung and chest complaints were rife. And then there was the ever-present stench of open sewage, rubbish, animal dung etc. In fact, the stench was so bad in 1858, the British parliament was suspended so members could go home and try to find relief behind closed doors. It became known as "The Great Stink."

LACK OF BREASTFEEDING

Infant formulas – albeit poor quality ones – were introduced in the mid-1800's, and over the next 100 years, breastfeeding rates dropped to just 25%. Not only did millions of babies miss out on the nurturing of their mother's breast, but their formula was poor quality, and often made with contaminated water in unsterile bottles. It's hardly a wonder that so many babies succumbed to diarrheal infections, such as typhoid fever. **(Diarrhea is simply the body flushing out toxic material, you do not die from this process you die from dehydration as the body would be assaulted with MORE toxic waste in the water given which would also have to be flushed out. Typhoid is not a contagious disease it is a toxic poisoning).**

IMPROPER GARBAGE DISPOSAL

Alleys and courtyards became littered with rubbish and waste, sometimes knee-high, which was not only offensive-smelling, but a great attraction for rats, pigs, dogs, cockroaches and swarms of flies. **(None of which would cause any disease to humans, they are in fact trying to clean up the environment).**

ANIMALS

Because horses and donkeys were used to transport goods, they also had to be housed in overcrowded cities, often in close quarters to humans, since space was at a premium. Rotting carcasses were left to decompose where they lay. Animal poo was a constant feature of the city streets. Pigs roamed freely in the streets, ferreting amongst the rubbish – some towns recorded more resident pigs than people. Animal slaughterhouses were located in amongst high-density tenement housing – animals were constantly slaughtered in full view of the surrounding residents, and the sounds and smell of death were constantly in the air. **(Again the proximity of animals with humans is not a cause of disease otherwise there would be the same deaths on farms as in towns which was not the case, in fact the very opposite).**

LACK OF CLEANLINESS

With less than 2% of the urban population with running water to their homes, and soap/detergents being expensive, washing of hands, clothes, plates and utensils was often done with dirty, recycled water, or not at all. And what about all the cloth diapers and sanitary pads? **(Hygiene in its proper sense has nothing to do with washing off germs. Bacteria are not killed by soap, what IS washed off are toxic chemicals and pollutants which are also present in the waste products of poisoned humans).**

MALNUTRITION

Millions of families subsisted on the cheapest food possible, sometimes only eating a meal every second day. Malnutrition was rife. **(Malnutrition is not the same thing as starvation so not eating every day should not be a problem as fasting is evidence of (except in growing children). It is more to do with WHAT is eaten, not how much)**. For example, at the turn of the 20th century, an estimated 1 in 2 children were suffering from rickets. In young girls, this often led to deformed hips, which then led to problems in childbirth, at a later date. With so little fresh fruits and vegetables in the diet, scurvy **(vitamin C deficiency)** also claimed many lives – an estimated 10,000 men during the California Gold Rush in the mid-1800's. Even in those who did not have scurvy, a mild deficiency in vitamin C must have been prevalent, *leading to weakened immunity* *to disease and infection.*

(The last sentence (in italics) is totally unnecessary and false. Scurvy was never an infectious disease, it was always malnutrition which in itself causes 'dis-ease'. There is no such thing as immunity from anything. Deaths were inevitable from the insane treatments meted out as shown in the next paragraph).

BAD MEDICINE

If you thought blood-letting and leeches were dubious enough, how about an injection of arsenic – proudly brought to you by Merck and Co? Or a gargle with mercury – where's the harm? And if you have smallpox, we'll dab your sores with corrosives…you know, to kill germs. **(LOL he's getting it now).** It's highly possible **(no it's absolutely definite)** that the medical 'treatments' killed more people than the diseases they were intended to treat **(sounds like the modern cancer industry).** Hospitals were known to be breeding-grounds **(breeding grounds of toxic drugs more like)** of disease, and in some cases, over-run by rats that were known to feed on patients. **(Delightful, so people were eaten alive in their beds then!).**

MENTAL AND EMOTIONAL STRESS

We now know that stress takes a huge toll on the immune system. **(Again no, there is no 'immune system'. Stress alone puts the body into a perpetual fight or flight mode which depletes the body of energy and halts any detox program until the stress is halted).** Can you imagine the mental anguish of being surrounded by abject poverty, and seeing no way of escape for yourself or your children? Or the panic of watching everybody you love succumb to a dreaded disease, and not having the knowledge or means to protect yourself? Or the dreariness of having absolutely nothing beautiful to look at, or any small comfort to make life more bearable? Not to mention the stress of toiling for long hours in monotonous or dangerous work **(filling your body with toxic pollution)**, with hardly a piece of dry bread to fill your hungry stomach?

Note that lack of vaccines is not on the list? **(AHA, now we get down to it).** That is because vaccines did not save us from diseases like you have been led to believe. See, it wasn't so much that the diseases were killers on their own, but the horrendous living conditions made them so. **(Oh dear, so the germs are more deadly when they live in bad conditions? That's just silly. There is no need to add another invisible entity to be a scapegoat here).** People simply couldn't keep up their defenses against such a constant onslaught. **(Their defenses being the ability to detox the constant onslaught of toxins?).**

Researchers [McKinley & McKinley] carefully analyzed all the data from 1900 to the 1970's and came to the conclusion that all medical advancements combined [which includes vaccination, and the discovery of penicillin, among other things] could only account for 3.7% of the decrease in deaths from infectious diseases. If they went back further, into the 1800's, that figure would be even less impressive…

We can thank toilets and plumbers and cars and fridges and fruit and town planners and clean water, and so forth, for the other 96.3% decrease in mortality from *infectious diseases*. **(No proof of any infectious diseases so far here, just toxic environments and malnourishment).**

Addendum

I've just been given some new information regarding smallpox which I think would go well here. Jim West commented: **"Smallpox is likely arsenic poisoning (symptoms are same) and the vax/Indian stories are a coverup. Smallpox was everywhere that European trappers or solders ventured. They all carried arsenic trioxide for tanning or perhaps hidden upstream warfare."**

I'm not sure I would class the vaxxing as a 'cover-up' per se maybe just an added toxic assault to tip the scales. So there is another reason to dismiss their contagion propaganda. It could maybe go in the 'contaminated' section but it also could be in a section of its own called **POISONING**.

CONTAGION – A FAIRY STORY

This was posted in a terrain theory group by Daniel Roytas; it was such a well put together post it deserves saving for posterity.

*This post contains scientific references of many studies that were undertaken to try and prove that germs cause disease.

All of the studies failed.*

Where is the evidence that viruses cause disease? I have been asking for almost 12 months now, and no one has been able to provide me with a single peer reviewed journal article showing an isolated virus causes disease. It should be so easy to look through the literature and find a study in a couple of minutes, yet no one seems to be able to do such a thing. Scientists and doctors have already done countless experiments to try and prove germ theory over the course of 120+ years, and all have failed.

So I will ask again, can anyone provide me one such study, showing an isolated virus causes disease in humans? If so, I will gladly stand corrected and recount everything I have ever said on this matter. There needs to be a truly scientific and intellectually honest conversation about this. This is the beauty of the scientific method, that we can ask questions, challenge our beliefs, put forward new ideas (that may or may not be correct) and learn new things. Here are just some of the experiments that have been done on the common cold/flu. Many studies like this have been done in other diseases like measles and chicken pox as well, and they have not been able to prove viral causation or contagion.

In March of 1919 Rosenau & Keegan conducted 9 separate experiments in a group of 49 healthy men, to prove contagion. In all 9 experiments, 0/49 men became sick after being exposed to sick people or the bodily fluids of sick people.

In November 1919, 8 separate experiments were conducted by Rosenau et al. in a group of 62 men trying to prove that influenza is contagious and causes disease. In all 8 experiments, 0/62 men became sick. Another set of 8 experiments were undertaken in December of 1919 by McCoy et al. in 50 men to try and prove contagion. Once again, all 8 experiments failed to prove people with influenza, or their bodily fluids cause illness. 0/50 men became sick. In 1919, Wahl et al. conducted 3 separate experiments to infect 6 healthy men with influenza by exposing them to mucous secretions and lung tissue from sick people. 0/6 men contracted influenza in any of the three studies. [21]

In 1920, Schmidt et al conducted two controlled experiments, exposing healthy people to the bodily fluids of sick people. Of 196 people exposed to the mucous secretions of sick people, 21 (10.7%) developed colds and three developed grippe (1.5%). In the second

---

[21] www.jstor.org/stable/30082102?seq=1...

group, of the 84 healthy people exposed to mucous secretions of sick people, five developed grippe (5.9%) and four colds (4.7%). Of forty-three controls who had been inoculated with sterile physiological salt solutions eight (18.6%) developed colds. **A higher percentage of people got sick after being exposed to saline compared to those being exposed to the 'virus'.** [22]

In 1921, Williams et al. tried to experimentally infect 45 healthy men with the common cold and influenza, by exposing them to mucous secretions from sick people. 0/45 became ill. [23]

In 1924, Robertson & Groves exposed 100 healthy individuals to the bodily secretions from 16 different people suffering from influenza. The authors concluded that 0/100 became sick as a result of being exposed to the bodily secretions. [24]

In 1930, Dochez et al. attempted to infect a group of men experimentally with the common cold. The authors stated in their results, something that is nothing short of amazing. **"It was apparent very early that this individual was more or less unreliable and from the start it was possible to keep him in the dark regarding our procedure. He had inconspicuous symptoms after his test injection of sterile broth and no more striking results from the cold filtrate, until an assistant, on the second day after injection, inadvertently referred to this failure to contract a cold. That evening and night the subject reported severe symptomatology, including sneezing, cough, sore throat and stuffiness in the nose. The next morning he was told that he had been misinformed in regard to the nature of the filtrate and his symptoms subsided within the hour. It is important to note that there was an entire absence of objective pathological changes."** [25]

In 1940, Burnet and Foley tried to experimentally infect 15 university students with influenza. The authors concluded their experiment was a failure. [26]

---

[22] www.pubmed.ncbi.nlm.nih.gov/19869857/
https://catalog.hathitrust.org/Record/102609951
[23] www.pubmed.ncbi.nlm.nih.gov/19869857/
[24] https://fakeologist.com/experiments-prove-sickness-is-not-contagious/
[25] www.pubmed.ncbi.nlm.nih.gov/19869798/
[26] onlinelibrary.wiley.com/.../j.1326-5377.1940...

Addendum

One question that frequently comes up is the old story of giving 'infected blankets' to the Native Americans to kill them. This story is a cover-up for the real killer which was again allopathic medicine and their vaccines. The proof is in plain sight as always. They vaccinated them. They got sick from the poisoning and died.

> The **Indian Vaccination Act** is a US federal law was passed by the US Congress in 1832.[1] The purpose of the act was to vaccinate the Indian Americans against smallpox to prevent the spread of the disease. Smallpox outbreaks were interfering with the removal of Native Americans from their land.[2] Vaccinating them would make it easier for the government to move them west, so white Americans could take their land.[3][4]

Read between the lines…"vaccinating them would make it easier to"… get rid of them.

Another little gem of an addendum I found on FB:

"That which can be asserted without evidence can be dismissed without evidence. The onus is on those making the claims that viruses exist to prove they exist."

I just finished reading all the books of **Charles Fort** (where we get the word 'Fortean' from) and he wrote this about germ theory. Keep in mind governments have known for over 200 years that the germ theory is false:

"Of all germ-distributors, the most notorious was Dr Arthur W. Waite, who, in the year 1916, was an embarrassment to medical science. In his bacteriological laboratory, he had billions of germs. Waite planned to kill his father-in-law, John E. Peck, 435 Riverside Drive, New York City. He fed the old man germs of diphtheria, but got no results. He induced Peck to use a nasal spray, in which he had planted colonies of the germs of tuberculosis. Not a cough. He fed the old man calomel to weaken his resistance. He turned loose hordes of germs of typhoid, and then influenza. In desperation, he lost all standing in the annals of distinctive crimes, and went common, or used arsenic. The old-fashioned method was a success. One's impression is that, if anything, diets and inhalations of germs may be healthful."

All these experiments seem like a long time ago, maybe they gave up trying to prove germ theory so thought it worth adding this little gem which happened during the whole AIDS plandemic (yup that was fake too).

December 7th 1994, Hollywood Roosevelt Hotel, Greensboro, N.C., Dr Willner (a medical doctor of 40 years' experience) an outspoken whistleblower of the AIDS hoax. In front of a gathering of about 30 alternative-medicine practitioners and several journalists, Willner stuck a needle in the finger of Andres, 27, a Fort Lauderdale student who says he has tested positive for HIV. Then, wincing, the 65-year-old doctor stuck it in himself. In 1993, Dr. Willner stunned Spain by inoculating himself with the blood of Pedro Tocino, an HIV positive hemophiliac. This demonstration of devotion to the truth and the Hippocratic Oath he took, nearly 40 years before, was reported on the front page of every major newspaper in Spain. His appearance on Spain's most popular television show evoked a 4 to 1 response by the viewing audience in favor of his position against the 'AIDS hypothesis.'

When asked why he would put his life on the line to make a point, Dr. Willner replied:

"I do this to put a stop to the greatest murderous fraud in medical history. By injecting myself with HIV positive blood, I am proving the point as Dr. Walter Reed did to prove the truth about yellow fever. In this way it is my hope to expose the truth about HIV in the interest of all mankind."

He tested negative multiple times.

Dr. Willner died of a heart attack 4 months later on 15th April 1995 (yeh right, funny how these naysayers all die suddenly).

Watch the video on YouTube of Dr Willner injecting HIV into himself. [27]

THE CORONA PHANTOM AND
WHAT IF THE VIRUSES DON'T EXIST?

DR. STEFAN LANKA 12.01.2021
(Translated by Tracey Northern & John Blaid)

Three ways I recommend for understanding and exploring the Corona crisis phenomenon.

---

[27] https://youtu.be/9WFhw5HHHbQ

THE FIRST way is to refute the virologists who make the claims that viruses are disease-causing through studying and exposing their papers. You will find that the statements and actions of the virologists are extremely unscientific. The photos, which allegedly show disease-causing viruses, actually show typical cell structures or artificial protein-fat-soap globules that are created when such mixtures are swirled around. With these photos it is crucial to know that the structures shown have never been characterized biochemically. In the structures shown, which are supposed to represent viruses, the long piece of genetic substance that they call the 'heart' of a virus, the genetic strand or the genome was never discovered or even searched for.

What is actually done when they claim the existence of a disease-causing virus is to mix very short pieces of gene sequences from a human, microbial and/or biochemical metabolism to construct a very long piece of genetic sequence, which would never really exist in nature.

Furthermore, little more than 50% of the gene sequences used here are real, i.e. originating from human and microbial metabolism. The remainder of the sequences required to form the 100% engineered gene sequence of the alleged viral genome are fictitious.

But it gets even better: The slightly more than 50% of the actually existing gene sequences that are used to construct a viral genome are themselves only a statistical average from an infinite and constantly changing variety of so-called gene sequences. In reality the metabolism produces constantly changing 'gene sequences', not a virus. These short 'nucleotides' serve to adapt to changes and are an essential process for survival in biological life.

New combinations of nucleotide sequences are constantly being made in every human being and every animal. If you look for short sequences of nucleotides that are similar to the 'gene sequences' that are reported as part of the virus, you will always find constant changes, which are touted as evidence of the mutation of the virus with no scientific proof. Such an alleged mutation of the corona virus – currently supposedly coming from England – is then used to tighten the restrictions, to cover up the effects of highly toxic corona 'treatments' and to include the symptoms of the immediate, medium and long-term vaccine damage caused by the highly toxic nano-particle and gene 'vaccinations' into the ever increasing definition of the syndrome 'Covid-19'.

Doubting and questioning is the first and most important obligation of every scientist. Anyone who calls this scientific questioning a conspiracy is being anti-scientific, antisocial and is a supporter of a superstition that must not be questioned.

Something that must not be questioned is always dangerous, manipulative and a basis for destruction and self-destruction. There is no need for a 'virus' as a cause of the visible destruction and self-destruction the corona panic measures bring. Here the historically grown and therefore unnoticed superstition in the minds of the majority of the population and a few good/bad high priests reinforced by the media is sufficient.

THE SECOND way I propose to find security and bearings is to study the story of where, why and how the idea arose that nature is evil and that there is an evil in its own right in biology. A materializing principle of evil ('cancer') that is able to wander inside the body ('metastases') and outside ('pathogens, viruses') cannot logically exist. Anyone who believes that 'cancer' is a malignant degeneration and does not know the real causes will also believe in flying mini-metastases in the form of invisible viruses.

As you walk through history, you will find that this good/bad materialism, which dominates today, emerged as a reaction to the generation of fear and abuse of power by religions in ancient Greece as a counter-reaction to centuries-long abuse of power by the churches. This materialism free of consciousness, spirit and soul became the basis of our Enlightenment and of biological and medical science.

Medicine and science were nationalized under this stipulation in 1858 and since then pseudoscience has been practiced almost exclusively in order to maintain the cellular pathology of Rudolf Virchow, which was not only refuted but never proven in 1858.

THE THIRD and probably the most helpful way for you to find your bearings and security is to learn superior explanations of life, health, disease and healing that have been emerging since 1981. Diseases are not theoretically triggered by pathogens or bad genes that inevitably result from the refuted theory of cellular pathology. Processes that we still wrongly view as independent diseases are triggered by events (such as a corona diagnosis) that affect the person concerned in an unexpected existential manner and actually isolate him or her from their environment.

Based on knowledge that has been documented a thousand times, it has been clearly proven that the assumptions and claims of an independent 'evil' does not exist in nature, in the body or in life. Biology cannot be good or bad. Biology simply is. The organism always behaves in a manner that enables survival even in extreme situations. For this purpose, the functions of the affected organs are usually increased. If that is not enough to escape from the life-threatening situation, either the tissue build-up or breakdown is increased in order to optimally adapt to the situation. Conventional medicine regards this as an independent disease that is supposedly triggered by defects, bad genes, poor immune functions, infections or a combination thereof.

If the triggering trauma is actually resolved or if the person succeeds in changing his relationship to it so that one can 'smile' at it again, the organism then tries to restore itself to its original state. Excess tissue is broken down or broken down tissue is rebuilt. Conventional medicine regards these processes as different diseases and consequently it is believed that each disease was triggered by another defect, an infection, etc.

From the perspective of today's 'medicine' (the doctrine of the suppression of symptoms by substances), what follows is misinterpreted as being independent of each other and as separate diseases in their own right:

1. The adaptation of the body to a permanent alarm from a trauma or a biological conflict.
2. The second phase, the healing phase after the practical or developed resolution of the trauma/biological conflict with the aim of restoring it to its original state.
3. In the switchover between the permanent alarm of the trauma phase and the healing process, healing crises occur which, depending on the duration and intensity of the biological conflict, can be more or less severe. These phenomena (sudden migraines, headaches, nerve pain, loss of sense of smell and orientation, dizziness, epilepsy, heart attack, pulmonary embolism, psychosis etc.) have been scientifically clarified, i.e. comprehensible, verifiable and predictable, which brings us to a causal and therefore functioning prophylaxis and therapy.

With this method of 'universal biology' (also well described by the ambiguous term 'Biology According to Hamer', since Dr. Ryke Geerd, Hamer removed the so-called evil from biology and medicine), expanded by the findings of nutritional science, Osteopathy, Physiology, Toxicology, Typology such as 'Terlusollogie', 'Human Design', (the sensational and documented findings of the Bruno Gröning circles) and other findings, all symptoms and particularly those of the constantly growing symptom complex 'Covid-19' can be explained without contradiction, without having to use the disproved assumptions of cell biology and the auxiliary hypotheses of infection, immune, gene and cancer hypotheses that necessarily result there from.

MD Ryke Geerd Hamer has clearly proven the complete reverse with his collection of knowledge (earlier as New Medicine, then as 'Medicina Sagrada', then as Germanic New Medicine and finally as Germanic Medicine or 'Germanic') in showing that every part of the body, every functional area of an organ represents a materialization of a unit of consciousness.

It can even be hit with a word to thus set off an alarm, even a fatal continuous alarm: "One word can kill", but also "One word can heal."

From this perspective, every unjustified generation of fear represents a kind of self-fulfilling prophecy that hits those people who believe in the existence and independence of materializing evil in the form of disease, disease genes, cancer, pathogens, viruses, etc. all the more. By observing and recognizing a meaningful and natural set of rules in biology, Dr Hamer has found the connection to the original philosophy of Ayurveda, in which the soul 'Atma' plays the decisive role. In the following, the various manifestations of metabolism (all bound to water) are taken into account.

Symptoms such as sudden headaches, loss of taste and sense of direction and dizziness are easily explained. They are all assigned to the 'Covid-19' list of symptoms, which has been growing steadily since the test was introduced. The original cause of the corona panic, was only the diagnosis of people with pneumonia, in whom no 'pathogens for pneumonia' were detectable (= atypical pneumonia).

Headaches, if they can be localized, are always due to a lack of oxygen, for example, if after the previous phase of a permanent alarm, in which the metabolism automatically switches from breathing to fermentation, is switched back to breathing, there is insufficient oxygen, or the oxygen cannot be transported or only with difficulty through the 'acidic' areas of the brain. The headache caused by the trigeminal nerve, which is in constant alarm, and headache caused by bleeding, among others, are explained in the specialist literature.

Dull headaches are caused, among other things, by the fact that the release of lactic acid and water, which has increased significantly during fermentation, cannot be removed, especially if the removal of water from the brain is restricted by a restriction of the cranio-sacral movements and/or by the kidneys.

The restriction of the sense of smell and the sense of direction (which is always linked to the sense of smell!) and the development of dizziness have also been clarified. Loss or impairment of the sense of smell and taste is often caused by swelling of the olfactory mucous membrane in the case of a cold. There are other possibilities that can lead to a loss of sense of smell.

From the findings of Universal Biology, a loss of sense of smell can also occur from a triggering event (shock) in which one does not want to smell something. You want to get rid of the danger (smell information) or even just a bad smell. 'Odor dangers' are experienced individually. It can be an actual danger, e.g. fire (smoke), or a danger that one experiences by association, e.g. the fictional virus. A face mask that has also been placed over the nose and emits an unpleasant odor can also lead to a loss of sense of smell. From the basis of Universal Biology, a loss of taste occurs through a triggering event that one does not want to taste/swallow. You want to get rid of the danger (taste information) or even just a bad taste.

The primary symptom on which the corona panic is based – pneumonia (always) represents a repair process, which in fact (always) can become critical. If panic, incorrect treatment, over treatment and/or various illnesses are added (= multimorbidity, as was and is the case in China, Italy, Germany and everywhere), the consequences can quickly be dramatic and fatal. It was never new.

See all available statistics before and during the Corona crisis.

Sources: The book 'Universal Biology After Aristotle, Kant and Hegel' by Richard Dien Winfield; the article by Ursula Stoll in the magazine Wissenschaft + (March 2020 about Corona and 'Covid-19 symptoms'); three contributions from me on a new perspective on life in issues 1, 2 and 3/2019 of Wissenschaft +. Valuable explanatory texts and statistics on the CoronaFakte Telegram channel.

Conclusion

When you have checked all of this, you will find that the corona crisis is nothing more than a self-perpetuating (predicted by me and others) completely irrational good/evil hysteria that bears no relation to scientifically provable biological reality.

Now you must decide whether the majority of the superstitious hysteria previously caused by the corona crisis will continue to destroy the foundations of biological, community and economic life or whether most people will emerge to rely on holism, reason and actual science, who will bring the corona crisis to repentance and out of 'good-bad think', acting and feeling toward a deeper understanding and thus knowing how to use it as an opportunity for everyone. [28]

CONTAGION – FACT CHECKED

So I've talked about the germ theory, how it was born and grew into the beast we are all supposed to live in fear of. I got some great feedback and just as I predicted the same question popped up, as it always does.

Don't get me wrong, I'm not knocking anyone for asking because I'm pretty sure I asked the same thing myself.

"WHAT ABOUT THE TIME WHEN WE ALL GOT CHICKENPOX/FLU/MEASLES?"

If it wasn't germs or viruses what was it?

So if you take away the germ theory what is left? QUESTIONS. A gaping hole that needs answers. Now I can't possibly speak to every case people will throw at me because there could be any number of reasons why people fall ill. They have to be looked at individually and personally. But to simplify matters, and I always like to simplify, we must stick to the rules we DO know are true.

YOU CAN ONLY BECOME SICK FOR 3 REASONS

1. **TOXEMIA** – Poisoning of any kind, it can be from pollution in the air and the water, even your food. It is drugs and especially vaccines. Poisoning is usually the main culprit being explained away with germ theory by claiming it's a contagious disease. A scapegoat for big industries.

2. **MALNUTRITION** – Does NOT mean starvation. Mal is French for BAD or WRONG. So eating the wrong diet basically. Being severely depleted in certain nutrients and remember all drugs (and poisons) deplete the body of nutrients as they get used up to deal with toxins. Particularly vitamin C it seems, which some claim might be a kind of chemical antidote or neutralizing agent which is why they have noticed it leaves the body so quickly. Remember that old Dr's saying about expensive urine?

3. **INJURY** – Physical or mental. Physical injury can be obvious, a cut or stab or a broken bone even bruises. It can also be

---

[28] Original German version:
www.bag-ivi-swissmedic-fall.ch/Corona_Phantom_13-1-2021.pdf

hidden as in internal injuries which could be caused by number 1 again (Toxemia), say, by swallowing a corrosive chemical or drugs like chemo and antibiotics which kill and injure our cells. Mental injury can also cause dis-ease, stress and shock being obvious and well documented. Ever heard a story of someone dying of a broken heart? And the old voodoo trick doctors use by telling someone they only have weeks to live? If you believe what doctors say you will comply and die when you've been told to. I wonder how many post mortems would reveal this if it was done properly and independently? ALL drugs have what they call 'side-effects'. These are also a kind of internal injury caused by poisoning which also depletes nutrients so a triple whammy.

Keeping these three things in mind and totally ignoring any germ theory nonsense we can go through all the big plagues and epidemics and look at them without tunnel vision. Let's look at them now in chronological order. I know it's a bit ridiculous given the time scale and lack of definitive proof but this first one has to be done as it's always brought up…

THE PLAGUE/BLACK DEATH

The Bubonic and Pneumonic plagues all seem to be lumped under the same umbrella...we are told roughly and varying numbers like 100-200 million died from it but to put it in perspective, it started in China (again yes) and supposedly spread right across Europe, the Middle East (and Africa eventually). This huge number is quoted even when they are only referring to the European plague.

BUT if you check the small print it was NOT one disease, it was many different diseases lumped under the same heading AND it covered 400 years. Some people have looked into the few written witness statements of the times and from them we get all manner of weird and wonderful stories. From aliens and spaceships, to bombs and flying fireballs in the skies to earthquakes, men in black and putrid smelling mists and fogs which killed crops and animals, not just people.

Look into it and all you will find are medieval conspiracy stories.

These earlier stories all seem to refer to Pneumonic symptoms meaning pneumonia and breathing problems and, if we take all the old writings at face value, were caused by sprayed poisons – but by who or what? We won't go there.

The Bubonic symptoms were completely different and were more like mumps and general swollen glands which points to more of an ingested poisoning rather than breathed in.

The rat fleas story which was jumped on later, has already been debunked and is not a contagion story anyway if it supposedly came from flea bites, that is not a contagion. But it didn't come from rat fleas anyway, according to modern computer models it couldn't have caused the disease to spread the way it appeared to.

The Bubonic version was said to follow the trade route called The Silk Road so we have rats and travelling tradesmen from China and Asia. What were they trading? China was already using the first version of vaccinations (variolation) which involved blowing powdered smallpox scabs (along with poisons no doubt), up the nose and was said to be 'crude and often fatal'. Yes I said smallpox scabs. Smallpox was an Asian disease at this time and hadn't hit Europe yet. Could they have been exporting this variolation practice and powders AND hence the appearance of a spreading disease? Seeing as it was picked up in Turkey years later by an English ambassador, Lady Mary Montagu, I would say it's highly likely. By then it had morphed into 'inoculation' by scratching the stuff into cuts instead of blowing it up the nose.

What other weird and wonderful {cough} dangerous herbal or chemical concoctions were being sold on the trade routes as medicines?

There was even a massive conspiracy theory in Europe that the Jews were poisoning wells to take over villages and small towns which resulted in the persecution and murder of Jews for years to come. There is even written evidence of a court case at the time of one particular Jewish merchant who claimed he was paid to do it. I'm not saying this was true but it has to be mentioned as it caused a lot of deaths and hoo-ha too at the time.

Nothing in any of the witness stories points to contagion though unless you are deaf dumb and blind to all the poisons being traded across the world, PLUS trying to find any coherent evidence and accurate dates and places is impossible.

To summarize, this was a lot of different diseases with varying causes spanning even more than 400 years .I spotted a book claiming the first case was in Constantinople in the year 592!! Basically we shouldn't even go there, it's all nonsense and we're supposed to be talking science here. But interesting to note the earliest vaccines were already spreading across the globe…

SCURVY

Scurvy WAS a contagious disease which killed many people over the years but sailors exposed its real cause eventually. In the 1500's a

French explorer accidentally cured his men of the scurvy with boiled pine leaves. They had no idea about vitamin C at the time but pine needles are full of it. So the lack of vitamin C or fresh fruit was not officially recognized at all.

It was left until the 19th century when British Naval Commander James Lind pioneered a program for making citrus foods available in all sea voyages. He also composed a book which described miracle cures encountered with the use of lemon juice. However, he was ignored for his advice which seemed loaded with speculations.

It wasn't until Captain Cook decided to try the limey cure 62 years later that the case was settled. If you look for symptoms of scurvy the list is long and very varied and there are pictures of rashes which look much like some kind of pox disease and lots of pics of rotten teeth. Just looking at them makes me want to reach for the fruit bowl.

Scurvy is an easy one, malnutrition and eventually toxemia from not being able to detox through lack of the right acids and not contagion at all and it only took them 200 years to work that one out. You can still see scurvy today, it's all around us, just look at all the people who don't eat their fruit. There's even an urban myth now that eating fruit rots your teeth – people are ridiculous sometimes.

SMALLPOX

Smallpox is always linked to the industrial revolution. It affected mostly city dwellers and industrial towns. Pollution was rife, the air was contaminated with all manner of poisonous gases and chemicals which also rained down on people like acid rain. There is no doubt in my mind this was an occupational disease caused by exposure to the noxious chemicals used in all the growing industries. Not only was it raining down from all the factory chimneys but workers were coming home covered in God knows what and getting into bed with their wives and children who all lived in squalor. Children were also put to work in the factories from a young age.

You can read all about the many diseases and symptoms caused by industry in a book called 'Diseases of Occupation and Vocational Hygiene' by George M. Kober.

It was noted at the time by Jenner (the father of vaccination) that milkmaids did not get smallpox because they'd had cowpox. I've heard theories online that it was because they drank milk but everyone else drank milk too though it had formaldehyde added to it for the townies to hide the sour taste as it went off. So it was more likely because they lived in the countryside where they had fresh air and fresh food. Food in cities and towns was not so fresh or cheap but often putrid. Few could afford the good stuff.

Treatments for smallpox were also of course extremely toxic, yes they smothered you in toxic/caustic chemicals to 'kill the bugs'. Similar was applied to bedding to kill bedbugs which they thought was causing it too. Did they mistake flea bites for smallpox? Probably in some cases.

Edward Jenner (a Freemason) invented the first vaccine for smallpox, basing his theory on the variolation technique imported from Turkey and his milkmaid cowpox theory. (The milkmaid story turned out to be a myth too, just a milkmaid's tale, pure hearsay).

Eleanor McBean pointed out in the 1950's in her book 'The Poisoned Needle' that cowpox is actually bovine syphilis. Jenner was injecting pus from cow syphilis sores into people to prevent them getting smallpox, and doctors with brains believe this crap.

Smallpox took off big time once the vaccines started rolling out and rates sky-rocketed. More people died after vaccines than did before them.

In 1871-2, England, with 98% of the population aged between 2 and 50 vaccinated against smallpox, experienced its worst ever smallpox outbreak with 45,000 deaths. During the same period in Germany, with a vaccination rate of 96%, there were over 125,000 deaths from smallpox.

The Leicester Experiment proved it was the vaccines causing deaths after they quarantined themselves (yes the whole city) and refused the mandatory vaccine. They had the lowest smallpox case and death rate in the whole of England. A similar experiment was done in America with same results.

Smallpox was never 'eradicated' if we look at it from a symptomology perspective; chickenpox, monkey pox, any pox, measles, hives and any skin based detox can be lumped in as the pox just with varying degrees of severity. If we apply the 3 rules and ignore germ theory, smallpox is poisoning of the skin (possibly misdiagnosis too) but also would have to include malnutrition, internal poisoning from poisons in food and water and then there was also the stress of awful living conditions – even bed bugs were implicated.

TUBERCULOSIS

Just like smallpox, TB was rife, especially amongst industrial workers and towns where air pollution was extremely toxic. There was even talk amongst doctors of an 'immunity' to the gases in workers exposed to them for long periods. Could that be the body giving up trying to detox as the mortality rate was still high despite no symptoms?

TB was also strongly linked to the smallpox vaccine, the excuse being some of the vaccines were 'contaminated' with TB by accident. That was obviously a red herring.

In the 1970's a tuberculosis vaccine trial in India involving 260,000 people revealed that more cases of TB occurred in the vaccinated than the unvaccinated. (The Lancet 12/01/80 page 73).

TB is also still linked today with rough living conditions and is rife among dairy cows but, instead of blaming the stressful and over medicated AND vaccinated life of dairy cows, the germ theory protagonists like to blame the poor and innocent badgers for the sickness, just because, like germs, they are in the vicinity.

TB has always been a general chronic running down of the body which is why it is seen nowadays in the homeless who are often (but not always) addicted to one drug or another.

It's believed to be caused by a bacteria called Tuberculin but in the late 1800's Mr. Koch found to his dismay that the bacteria was rife in healthy people and not always there in sick people so could not be the cause yet they still blame it to this day.

With no proof it is contagious it has to be a lifestyle disease again with multiple causes, all three in fact, malnutrition, poisoning and stress.

SPANISH FLU

This disease did not spread outwards in all directions like a contagious disease should, it popped up almost simultaneously in several army barracks amongst soldiers. Coincidentally, in preparation for WW1, a massive military vaccination experiment involving numerous prior developed vaccines took place in Fort Riley, Kansas where the first 'Spanish Flu' case was reported. [29]

One of the startling things they said about the disease was how it seemed to knock the young and fit the hardest. Like soldiers? And that it would be fast, like one day fit and healthy, the next day dead. Sort of like as if they'd been poisoned!! The fledgling pharmaceutical industry, sponsored by the 'Rockefeller Institute for Medical Research', had something they never had before – a large supply of human test subjects.

Supplied by the U.S. military's first draft, the test pool of subjects

---

[29] www.ncbi.nlm.nih.gov/pmc/articles/PMC2126288/pdf/449.pdf

ballooned to over 6 million men.

From January 21-June 4, 1918, an experimental bacterial meningitis vaccine cultured in horses by the Rockefeller Institute for Medical Research in New York was injected into soldiers at Fort Riley. They had around 6 MILLION soldiers to experiment on. WW1 U.S. soldiers were given 14–25 untested, experimental vaccines within days of each other, which triggered intensified cases of ALL the diseases at once. They decided to reclassify this as a new disease (Spanish Flu).

How did all the people at home start dying when the soldiers came home if it wasn't contagious? Answer – well they didn't want them to catch it so they vaccinated them too.

An American called Eleanor McBean whose parents were doctors at the time, wrote that **"only the vaccinated died"**. Her unvaccinated parents caught nothing from the sick people they treated.

Another culprit seems to be the newly invented wonder drug ASPIRIN. People were given doses as high as 400 times the lethal dose we use today as soon as they showed symptoms. There was of course hysteria going on in the UK surrounding the news of deaths from a new contagious disease, plus soldiers already suffering post-traumatic stress were committing suicide and even murder in their madness. Even this madness was blamed on the flu, not the war.

Treatments in UK were ridiculous too. I found this interesting snippet on a BBC article.

Viruses were not well understood at the time and doctors were at a loss as to how to treat people.

"'Cures' ranged from standard camphor and quinine to alcohol - whisky in particular was sworn as the cure," said Ms Mawdsley.

"But some more extreme cures like creosote and strychnine were used. Basically, people were so desperate they would try anything."

Err, viruses hadn't been invented yet luv.

Autopsies after the war proved that the 1918 flu was NOT a 'FLU' at all. It was caused by random dosages of an experimental 'bacterial meningitis vaccine', which to this day mimics flu-like symptoms. The massive, multiple assaults with additional vaccines on the unprepared immune systems of soldiers and civilians created a 'killing field.' Those that were not vaccinated were not affected.

So yet again it seems vaccines and drugs were the cause of this 'plague' – maybe add in a splash of injury and stress from the war too.

POLIO

The pro-vaxxers favourite poster plague and the easiest to debunk. Polio cropped up around orchards which had been sprayed with arsenic as a pesticide to kill bugs which might spoil the apples. The same thing happened when a new colour (Paris Green) became the rage and was added to paints and wallpapers with the secret ingredient arsenic.

Originally polio was classified as any paralysis of parts of the body. Nurse/Sister Kenny demonstrated to doctors and the world that it wasn't necessarily a paralysis at all but a muscle spasm and treated it with massage and heat packs successfully. She was ignored of course. They didn't want that sort of cure.

Symptoms called polio always followed pesticide use. DDT was the next big one after they banned the old arsenic. It was hailed as a cure-all and sprayed freely on children and public spaces like swimming baths.

We've all heard the tales of kids 'catching polio' after visiting the pool but no-one put 2 and 2 together, or maybe they did coz hey, money to be made. So along came the vaccines which first off killed more kids than the swimming pools did.

Look up THE CUTTER INCIDENT. Then another vaccine with, at the same time, a NEW DEFINITION OF POLIO.

Because people were still getting the same symptoms which couldn't possibly BE polio after vaccination they decided to say they had meningitis instead.

When I first heard this I had to find proof and went to look at the old CDC stats and sure enough, the year of the Salk vaccine the numbers for meningitis and polio swap over exactly. Saw it with my own eyes. No doubt it's gone now from the web but there is still evidence of these stat swaps, thanks to the Waybackmachine.

Sample Months	Reported Cases of Polio	Reported Cases of Aseptic Meningitis
July 1955 (Before the new polio definition was introduced.)	273	50
July 1961 (After the new polio definition was introduced.)	65	161
September 1966 (After the new polio definition was introduced.)	5	256

Cases of polio were more often reported as aseptic meningitis after the vaccine was introduced, skewing efficacy rates.

Source: The Los Angeles County Health Index: Morbidity and Mortality, Reportable Diseases.

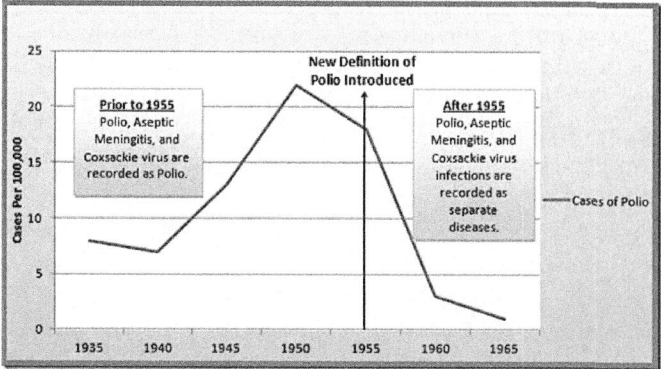

In 1977, Dr Jonas Salk, who developed the first polio vaccine, testified along with other scientists that mass inoculation against polio was the cause of most polio cases throughout the USA since 1961.

So ignoring the unproven contagious notion, it's safe to say polio is a poisoning specifically of the nervous system caused by nerve poisons which coincidentally are also an ingredient in most vaccines. Polio was never eradicated as many after-effects of vaccines are the same thing given a new name.

They even made vaccines for the new names for the same disease. Like Meningitis B and now the MenACWY. Clever eh!

Some of the new polio names include Guillain Barre, MS, ME, Meningitis (all forms), ALS, Transverse Myelitis, Bell's Palsy, non-paralytic polio, etc. etc. ANY vaccine can cause polio-like symptoms which they will never call polio.

HIV/AIDS

You could say this one plandemic was the one which started us all questioning the existence of all viruses because there were ructions going on in the science world over who had discovered the HI virus or even if they had at all. It also turned the immune theory on its head which should have been a mistake that exposed all their theories by stating that the presence of antibodies meant you HAD HIV not that you were IMMUNE to it. The disease it's meant to cause (AIDS) was first seen in the gay community of Los Angeles where the men were presenting to doctors with sick livers (hepatitis) from all the alcohol and drugs they took. Doctors then added antibiotics to the mix for the perceived STD's but the real stinger came when they tested out a new vaccine for Hepatitis B on the community.

After the vaccine their whole bodies seemed to shut down which they claimed was an immune system shut down so called it AIDS. "Acquired Immunodeficiency Syndrome" Where was it 'acquired' from? Couldn't possibly be the new vaccine on trial could it? Nooooo. Where did they follow up those trials and where did AIDS next reappear? Yeh Africa. Big pHarma's favourite playground full of human guinea pigs. What do they use to test if you have HIV? The PCR test.

Just like now with covaids it can find any genetic sequence they want to find in anyone at any time if they do enough cycles. Even its inventor was screaming from the hilltops that this was scientific fraud. So what happens if you get a positive test for HIV AND you are gay? They prescribe a failed chemo drug AZT (killed too many cancer patients) and voila, you have a new victim whose whole body shuts down from systemic poisoning. AIDS is death by poisoning. The HI virus does not exist, it was never isolated, Gallo lied.

Fauci was also involved in that scam.

Interestingly, in 1990, a UK survey involving 598 doctors revealed that over 50% of them refused to have the Hepatitis B vaccine despite belonging to the high risk group urged to be vaccinated. [30]

One big change that came with the AIDS scare was the hyping of condoms laced with chemical spermicides (another pesticide) which I personally suspect caused another manufactured and over diagnosed epidemic called cervical cancer, which they've also managed to invent a new scapegoat virus for (HPV sounds a lot like HIV) AND a new vaccine. Wow, the money train just keeps rolling on down the track...

COVAIDS-19

The so-called novel disease was first reported in China (just like the very first plague we talked about). It caused breathing difficulties in Wuhan, the most polluted city in the world, for which everyone wore masks already. Phew, good to know those masks really worked huh!

No covid virus to date has been isolated, classified and put through Kochs Postulates. No virus. "So what is killing people?" is the question everyone asks at this point. It's pretty obvious what killed the original

---

[30] British Med Journal, 27/1/1990

victims but there's another ingredient which no-one mentioned except one financial news website. See chapter 'Something You Should Know'.

China had also just vaccinated its population with a new experimental SARS vaccine. Yup you heard that right. Another cover-up for the vaccines? Seeing a pattern yet? Next stop was Italy, also in an area where they'd just mandated a new vaccine for the old folks PLUS the usual flu vaccine.

Then it seemed to jump to New York where for the past year they have been mandating vaccines too. Again, all these cities were highly polluted areas not only with your usual pollution but now the EMF pollution was being pushed to new heights with test roll-outs of 5G. All the big headline areas have these 3 things in common. No telling which of the 3 is the scapegoat for which of the other 3, it's all just a mass confusion and no-one is looking at anything because it's been decided it's a virus. After the 3 main cities reported this novel illness it probably might have fizzled out so they just added lists of more and more symptoms which they claimed were all covid, so transferring anyone with a sniff or a cough into the covid bracket along with those PCR tests set to give out mostly positive results, until BINGO they have manufactured a pandemic. What's the only thing that can stop this now? Another bloody vaccine of course. This story is getting so tediously predictable now.

I gave you a snippet from the experiments done to PROVE contagion in the 'Germ Theory' chapter. After every one of them failed to show any disease being passed person to person no more have been done since 1940. Not one person caught anything. Here's two more snippets – just to hammer it home some more...

1. In 1937 Burnet & Lush conducted an experiment exposing 200 healthy people to bodily secretions from people infected with influenza. 0/200 became sick.

2. In 1940, Burnet and Foley tried to experimentally infect 15 university students with influenza. The authors concluded their experiment was a failure. [31]

---

[31] https://onlinelibrary.wiley.com/doi/abs/10.5694/j.1326-5377.1940.tb79929.x

www.ncbi.nlm.nih.gov/pmc/articles/PMC2065253/?page=9&fbclid=IwAR3iH7vkzc6YWodurQhf3OfCn_0l4keB5IpQLg0TELcbb9jp04qDqDt4vLo

True causes will never be investigated as long as everything is focused on this notion of flying viruses and contagion. We can never get to the bottom of it if we don't investigate toxic chemicals and drugs but the science of toxicology has been completely side-lined by virology. No-one will go there, it's almost like it's got some deadly contagious disease. A disease called truth maybe.

Now we're faced with a new kind of pollution to contend with which no-one is even allowed to point at for fear of being banned from the internet. EMF's. Electromagnetic Frequencies. With that we are entering the realms of physics and other sciences which I am not as read-up on yet. I can recommend the book 'The Invisible Rainbow' by Arthur Firstenberg though.

EMF's have also been implicated in the Spanish Flu as it was when radio was first used, but I think we have enough evidence from then we don't need to rake up more, it's just another puzzle piece to keep an eye on.

I've written several articles on some of the diseases we've talked about here which all link to this contagion topic so have included links for further information and sources if you want to dig deeper. Just try to keep the only three reasons in your mind while thinking about specific illnesses (toxins, malnutrition and physical or mental injury) and you can't go wrong. If the mainstream are all pointing us in one direction you know there is something behind their backs they don't want you to see.

I hope what I've told you here will help to get rid of the fear of contagion and steer you towards the real villains in this story, the poison creators who are careful not to take their own medicines, the liars and deceivers who run the world and the media who sell us the lies and poisons.

We are not contagious vectors, there is no such thing as an 'asymptomatic carrier'. You cannot catch disease just like you cannot catch health. A fear which prevents you from living could actually be the death of you if you carry on believing this nonsense so go hug someone and let's get back to living instead of just surviving.

"...all Compulsory Vaccination should immediately be abolished, and that its continuation, with these proofs against it, would be a most gross medical blunder and malpractice and a grave violation of the basic American principle of Inherent Individual Rights, in being a serious menace to human health and life, a frequent cause of wide-spread epidemics and

demonstrably more fatal in many instances than natural disease itself, and therefore a shocking violation of all true medical ethics and a disgrace alike to modern medicine and. Modern legislation which should no longer tolerate the practice."

– Quote from Chas. M. Higgins, December 1919

My friend **Dawn Lester, co-author of the book 'What Really Makes You Ill?'**, has written an excellent article which will fill in any holes that I've left. Here's a couple of snippets from her article:

"It is interesting to note that the origin of the word 'contagion' is the Latin contagio, which only refers to direct contact. But, as the Merriam Webster definition shows, it is now regarded as involving indirect as well as direct contact. This of course allows the medical establishment to claim that so-called 'infectious agents' can spread through the air or through indirect contact by people touching the same surfaces, despite the fact that none of these modes of transmission have been proven scientifically to occur. This change of meaning has also enabled the medical establishment to use the words infection and contagion virtually interchangeably, even though this does not reflect their original meaning."

"Unfortunately, as we discuss in detail in our book, What Really Makes You Ill, the medical establishment operates from the basis of a flawed understanding of 'disease', which is not an entity that attacks the body indiscriminately to cause the symptoms of illness. Instead, the symptoms associated with what are called 'infectious diseases' represent the body's efforts to expel toxins, repair damage and restore health. This is explained by Herbert Shelton in his book, Natural Hygiene: Man's Pristine Way of Life, in which he refers to 'acute disease' and states that this term refers to, "...vital action in some one or all of the living tissues or organs in resisting and expelling injurious substances and influences and in repairing damages."

The significance of this statement, which cannot be overstated, is that it demonstrates the true nature of 'disease' and the purpose of the symptoms produced by the body. It is therefore important to recognise that the symptoms each person experiences will be unique to them because of their unique exposures to the 'injurious substances and influences' that affect their bodies." [32]

* There's a video of this on The Crazz Files, if you want to listen *

[32] www.whatreallymakesyouill.com/contagion-infection-deceptive-appearances/

WHAT ARE PEOPLE DYING FROM?

After I wrote 'Ex-Spurts – Who Do You Listen To?' I got asked this:

"But how can we expect people to believe that there is no virus, when they've watched the surge of deaths within the period the virus was announced?" It's the same thing I hear over and over again and finally I think I have to address it.

I know it's been addressed over and over but the message still has not hit home, maybe because no-one has put all the evidence down in one place. There are lots of people shouting about various causes and figures and graphs galore giving opposing views. There is mostly skewed data which basically means they are not showing the whole picture. They can make a graph using real accurate data but then they may only show the tail end of the graph making it look like something it is not. This has been done throughout the history of vaccines and more recently with the famous hockey stick graphs of global warming.

Firstly to address this question was there really a 'surge in deaths' in 2020? To find this out we need to look at overall death figures with no confounding factors. Look at the World Death Rate from 1950 to 2023 for real figures. [33]

Edit: Due to online censorship it seems all the stats have been fiddled with or 'delayed'. Ask yourself why they would delay the figures for 2020 when they were giving death counts on the media day by day and week by week, unless they were trying to cover them up? Anyone with any info on unadulterated numbers please let me know.

A Johns Hopkins study said there were 'No Excess Deaths in 2020'.

"First, Johns Hopkins University, in an official newsletter, reported that by its independent review of CDC data, there are no excess deaths in 2020. Johns Hopkins is a pillar of the medical and academic establishments and has been one of the official voices on the Covid issue. The notion of excess deaths is at the foundation of the claim that there is a pandemic happening. Any other year, this scenario would have made headlines and there would have been follow-up by the national press corps. COVID-19 mainly affects the elderly and experts expected an increase in the percentage of deaths in older age groups. However, this increase is not seen from the CDC data. In fact, the percentages

[33] https://www.macrotrends.net/countries/WLD/world/death-rate

of deaths among all age groups remain relatively the same," the University published in its official newsletter.

"These data analyses suggest that in contrast to most people's assumptions, the number of deaths by COVID-19 is not alarming. In fact, it has relatively no effect on deaths in the United States," the article continues.

"This caused such an uproar that five days later, the administration tried to walk back the article, claiming it was issuing the retraction "to stop the spread of misinformation, as we noted on social media." They revert to the authority of the same CDC whose data the paper's authors analyzed, ignoring their own findings and declaring 300,000 dead Americans over the norm. "It is impossible to dismiss this as a conspiracy theory, or to say it's the result of some oversight. It was a statistical study by one of the most prestigious institutions in the world."

According to Chinese and international public health agencies, the epidemic started in Wuhan, in a hospital, with a single patient who had pneumonia. The doctors could find no cause. The city of Wuhan is famous for clouds of foul pollution. The unprecedented combination of toxic compounds in the air constitutes a clear and present danger. In summer 2019 there was a large protest in the city focusing on this very issue. Why would this patient be a mystery in the first place? Why would researchers look for a virus no one had ever seen before? The entire 'origin story' of the 'coronavirus epidemic' is riddled with exaggerations and fabrications. [34]

Finding traces of the virus in humans and then calling these people 'infected' and 'carriers' and 'spreaders' and 'epidemic cases' is ridiculous. To date NO VIRUS isolation has been performed, the original was faked and produced 'in silico' which means ON A COMPUTER. China has not reported a single Covid death since May 2020!

"I have been to China, I have seen in person how they will protest over something then the CCP says OMG, look, virus, then lock down the city and go in and arrest all the protesters, killing them, this was done in Wuhan, then once they are done, then the CCP said, all clear, no more virus, there was no more protesters,

---

[34] https://thediplomat.com/2019/07/environmental-protest-breaks-out-in-chinas-wuhan-city

they was all killed in the jail hospital that had 2 large incinerators running 24 hours a day, at the time on the world heat map you could zoom in on the jail hospital and see them operating in real time, China does this to avoid UN human rights violations, it's really just that simple, it's a cover story to hide mass murder, in Wuhan they were in fact protesting like mad, and yes people were dying from a lung infection, but, it was from 5 trash incinerators pumping out 10,000 tons of burnt trash per day. you see, the news media only tells you what they want you to see, or think, so if you do not know to look for the truth, you do not know you're being lied to." – Testimony of J. Parsons (Jan 2020)

So what was all the fuss about in Italy?

Early reports from a Swiss Doctor, Published March 14, 2020; Updated March 27, 2020:

A Swiss medical doctor provided the following information on the current situation in order to enable our readers to make a realistic risk assessment.

According to the latest data of the Italian National Health Institute ISS, the average age of the positively-tested (with the now discredited PCR test) deceased in Italy is currently about 81 years. 10% of the deceased are over 90 years old. 90% of the deceased are over 70 years old.

80% of the deceased had suffered from two or more chronic diseases. 50% of the deceased had suffered from three or more chronic diseases. The chronic diseases include in particular cardiovascular problems, diabetes, respiratory problems and cancer.

Less than 1% of the deceased were healthy persons, i.e. persons without pre-existing chronic diseases. Only about 30% of the deceased are women.

The Italian Institute of Health moreover distinguishes between those who died from the coronavirus and those who died with the coronavirus. In many cases it is not yet clear whether the persons died from the virus or from their pre-existing chronic diseases or from a combination of both.

The two Italians deceased under 40 years of age (both 39 years old) were a cancer patient and a diabetes patient with additional complications. In these cases, too, the exact cause of death was not yet clear.

The doctor also points out the following aspects: Northern Italy has one of the oldest populations and the worst air quality in Europe, which had already led to an increased number of respiratory diseases and deaths in the past and is likely an additional risk factor in the current epidemic.

The most important indicator for judging the danger of the disease is not the frequently reported number of positively-tested persons and deaths, but the number of persons actually and unexpectedly developing or dying from pneumonia (so-called excess mortality). EXACTLY!!

1.   Zhuang et al., potential false-positive rate among the asymptomatic infected individuals' in close contacts of COVID-19 patients, Chinese Medical Association Publishing House, March 2020.

2.   Grasselli et al., Critical Care Utilization for the COVID-19 Outbreak in Lombardy, JAMA, March 2020.

3.   WHO, Report of the WHO-China Joint Mission on Coronavirus Disease 2019, February 2020.

Important reference values include the number of annual flu deaths, which is up to 8,000 in Italy and up to 60,000 in the US; normal overall mortality, which in Italy is up to 2,000 deaths per day; and the average number of pneumonia cases per year, which in Italy is over 120,000.

Current all-cause mortality in Europe and in Italy is still normal or even below-average. Any excess mortality due to Covid-19 should become visible in the European monitoring charts (and it never did become visible).

Congressman V. Sgarbi of Italy: "25 thousand people did not die of the coronavirus in Italy… The 25 thousand dead, as Prof. Bassetti said, died of cancer and heart attacks, etc.… It's a way to terrorize Italians and impose a dictatorship!" (May 2020)

Some people, reading will say, "But what about all the people who are sick in this epidemic?" Take a step back. A so-called CONFIRMED CASE OF CONVID IS BASED PURELY ON PCR. Now 18 months in the CDC has confirmed what us 'conspiracy nuts' AND the bloody inventor of the 'test' said, that it cannot find a virus. Their explanation is it can't differentiate between the flu and covid, well that is because it only finds and amplifies bits of genetic code which it turns out can be found in anyone at any time if you just turn up the dial (cycles) on the test.

So the CDC is ditching the PCR. Which means we can go back and ditch ALL the 'cases' which have been propping up the case-demic.

"Thanks to mass-murderer Dr. Fauci, Remdesivir was the ONLY approved treatment for Covid-19 patients yet, up until then, had never been approved to treat anything and in every trial, it proved ineffective only causing more damage! Fauci knew the experimental drug Remdesivir was deadly, yet mandated it anyway. This dangerous drug poisoned people's kidneys, which caused their lungs to fill with fluid/mucus until they drowned or were put on ventilators that killed 97% of them. Likewise, during the 1980's Fauci discouraged and prevented inexpensive treatments for 'AIDS' while exclusively pushing AZT (Azidothymidine) – a failed chemotherapy drug that, like Remdesivir, was so extremely toxic and fatal that the inventor didn't even think it was worth patenting. This drug is what ultimately killed hundreds of thousands of AIDS patients, not HIV. Worth noting that both for-profit-mass-murder-by-pharmaceutical-drug schemes relied on the fraudulent misuse of the RT-PCR to diagnose a virus. With a track record like Fauci's, it should be no surprise when the death tally from the clot shots he's been pushing far exceeds the number of deaths from AZT, Remdesivir, and even that of WWII put together." [35]

    – **Jamey Scott Breinberg**

The Mysterious Death of Dr Fauci's Most Notable Critic. Kary B. Mullis, the 1993 Nobel Prize winning inventor of the Polymerase Chain Reaction process, explains why the PCR test cannot be used as a reliable medical diagnostic tool but can be used as a deceptive snake oil selling tool. A video on Bitchute also infers that his death, just months before the Coronavirus 'epidemic' was being rolled out into public awareness, was a suspiciously convenient event for the plandemic promoters. [36]

This is from a post I wrote on March 8th 2020:

Some worrying yet eye-opening statements from Dr Inglesby of Johns Hopkins University Hospital –

"Overall mortality of this disease is difficult to calculate because of the different ways we are DIAGNOSING the disease".

"The more we do diagnosis…the more that will drive down the

---

[35] https://principia-scientific.com/doctor-reveals-remdesivir-is-real-cause-of-covid-19-maladies/
[36] https://www.bitchute.com/video/yyX5k0Qq7O13

overall case fatality rate".

"We need to expand diagnostic testing".

"In China we've seen at least 20% have NO SYMPTOMS which makes containing the disease...particularly challenging".

(Body language – fiddles with pen and water bottle = stress).

The tests do NOT look for any virus therefore they cannot confirm evidence of a virus. Why the hots for these tests? A disease with NO SYMPTOMS is NOT A DISEASE!!!! This is insane. ALL the symptoms they said were 'coronavirus' were typical cold or flu symptoms but that wasn't enough for them so they kept adding more.

The so-called 'SARS-CoV-2' genetic material doesn't exist as a proven viral disease-causing pathogen. The COVID-19 'disease' is just any variety of symptoms pertaining to any number of known illnesses or medical conditions. The reported covid deaths are the mislabeled results of those other real disease causes.

How many people actually SAW someone they know die of covid, actually sat and held their hand while they passed away from COVID and nothing else?

Did you know that officially iatrogenic death is the number three killer in the Western world? That means death by medicine and they don't even count the deaths from chemo, radiation and statin drugs amongst the official stats. If we add those in instead of lying and lumping them under heart disease and cancer, doctors are the number one killer. Where does everyone die these days? Under the care of doctors.

This known fact was added to with the way they changed the whole protocol of hospital admissions. The PPE, the PCR testing and then the ridiculous panic treatment of inducing coma's and putting people onto ventilators therefore raising their chance of dying to 80%. Very few people recover from ventilation.

The old folks were also given a very hard time of it. Isolated from all their loved ones, alone and distressed they were basically starved to death, put on DNR notice, withheld water and now it turns out they were also drugged with a euthanizing drug called Midazolam.

Now we all know that all those old folks were already dying in the homes before any mention of covid BUT what is really sad is they were hurried along towards their demise and they died ALONE without their loved ones to say goodbye. That is criminal as well as genocide.

Despite all the insane cruelty to our old grandparents the actual death stats did not even blip. They were completely normal for that age range. So in answer to the other question (not sure it was a serious one), "Is The Death Merely As A Result Of Fear?"

I'm pretty sure fear played a big part in it yes, amongst other things…

Covid is Social 'Munchausen Syndrome' ('Factitious Disorder') Imposed Socially via Extensive-Intensive Media Propaganda and Coercive Social Reinforcement. Munchausen Syndrome is a mental disorder in which a person repeatedly and deliberately acts as if he or she has a physical or mental illness when he or she is not really sick. With covid, the disorder is imposed socially by the State and the monopolized corporate media and economic network (employers and commercial distributors), as well as by the infected carriers of the disorder themselves, colloquially known as 'Karen's' or 'Covidiots'.

If you do not believe people can die just through the power of the mind take a look at this gruesome experiment…

"My interest in the psychological was constantly rearoused by clinical observations and by studying the encyclopedic literature. A report in an Indian medical periodical "Killed by the Imagination"* left an indelible impression early in my career.

A Hindu physician was authorized by prison authorities to conduct an astonishing experiment on a criminal condemned to death by hanging. The doctor persuaded the prisoner to permit himself to be exsanguinated – bled to death – assuring him that death, though gradual, would be painless. The convict, on agreeing, was strapped to a bed and blindfolded. Vessels filled with water were hung at each of the four bedposts and set up to drip into basins on the floor. The skin on his four extremities was scratched, and the water began to drip into the containers, initially fast, then progressively slowing. By degrees the prisoner grew weaker, a condition reinforced by the physician's intoning in a lower and lower voice. Finally the silence was absolute as the dripping of water ceases. Although the prisoner was a healthy young man, at the completion of the experiement, when the water flow stopped, he appeared to have fainted. On examination, however, he was found to be dead despite not having lost a single drop of blood.

Over the centuries, a wealth of similar anecdotes has been amassed. The medical profession has long known that nervous activity influences every part of the body. Nearly 350 years ago, William Harvey, discoverer of the circulation of the blood, stated:

"Every affection of the mind that is attended with either pain or pleasure, hope or fear, is the cause of an agitation whose influence extends to the heart." *N.S. Yagwer "Emotions as a Cause of Rapid and Sudden Death" Archives of Neurology and Psychiatry 36 (1936).

– **From 'The Lost Art Of Healing' by Bernard Lown**

Ibn Sina (ca. 970-1037, Islamic philosopher and physician) explains the seriousness of stress and fear for human health:

"An epidemic was going to one of the cities. A man watched it and asked him: 'Where are you going, Epidemic? The epidemic replied: I go to this city to kill a thousand of its people. When the epidemic came out of the city, the man said to him: How hard you are! You killed twenty thousand people of the city! The epidemic replied: I only killed a thousand; the rest killed themselves by delusion and fear... Delusion is half the disease; reassurance is half the medicine."

There is a lot of speculation that death rates would spike because people were not able to get the 'treatment' they needed during lockdowns and hospital closures but from what we know of iatrogenic death I would have to disagree and say the death rates will probably fall as people are not being poisoned with pharmaceutical drugs, but we shall have to wait for those figures to prove me right.

All in all the actual death figures during this 'pandemic' have NOT CHANGED CONSIDERABLY, in fact they are lower than average therefore there could not BE any pandemic at all. People die, every day. Stop attributing their deaths to a fictitious virus. It is not on us to prove there is no virus, besides it's impossible to scientifically prove a negative. The onus is on YOU to prove there IS a virus.

Remember this quote from Christopher Hitchens?

"Forgotten were the elementary rules of logic, that extraordinary claims require extraordinary evidence and that what can be asserted without evidence can also be dismissed without evidence."

Been saying for a very long time that the aptly named invisible virus is more than likely just pneumonia reclassified.

Out of all the so-called covid deaths, covid-pneumonia was on the death certificate 1804 times out of 2156 reported.

When you dig deeper you can find other almost identical characteristics as covid. 550-1000 out of every 100000 people get CAP which is community acquired pneumonia of which around 1% die.

Then there are also two different types of pneumonia that are very commonly contracted in hospitals called hospital-acquired pneumonia and ventilator-associated pneumonia. Yes, two of the most common ways to get pneumonia are by being hospitalized and put on a ventilator. I wonder why they kept putting more and more on ventilators? Surely it's not to get the death rate up? Both affect mainly the older generation and when put on a ventilator or hospitalized mortality rates shoot up to 30% and as high as 70%. Sounds like the perfect candidate to create the illusion of a pandemic…don't you think?

Well this FOI request from James McCumiskey shows very strong evidence that could certainly be the case. Furthermore, the new type of pneumonia called covid-pneumonia doesn't even exist except for on death certificates as there is no official ICD code for covid-pneumonia, even though they have been using it for 16 months as a cause of death. The WHO just told them to classify it that way. Bit strange that.

FOI REQUEST

"I would like to request the total amount of deaths recorded as the cause of death for the following:

1. It is my understanding that a new classification of pneumonia came about this year called covid-pneumonia. Is that correct?

2. If so can you please provide stats for how many people have this as the cause of death from March 2020 in Northern Ireland.

3. Can you also provide how many people have died from pneumonia in each of the last 5 years in Northern Ireland?

4. And can you please provide how many people have died from the flu in each of the last 5 years in Northern Ireland?

5. Given that Ventilator-associated pneumonia (VAP) is a common nosocomial infection affecting up to 20% of patients admitted to intensive care units (ICUs) 1-3 VAP is associated with a 2-7-fold increased risk of death according to this BMJ article. Firstly why are you using ventilators to treat patients and secondly what are you doing to differentiate between covid-pneumonia and other types of pneumonia like VAP?

FOI RESPONSE

I can confirm the Department holds some of the information requested, however, FOI Exemption Section 21 (Information is accessible by other means) applies, as some of the information is reasonably accessible by other means. The Northern Ireland Statistics and Research Agency (NISRA) collates data on registrations of death.

1. Based on the WHO ICD-10 cause of death coding framework which is used to identify the underlying/main cause of death, there is no formal classification of covid-pneumonia therein. However, covid and pneumonia or covid-pneumonia has been referred to by medics when certifying deaths.

2. As there is no official ICD code for covid-pneumonia, a text search has been carried out where covid-pneumonia or covid and pneumonia appears anywhere on death certificates. From this analysis 1,804 cases were found since March 2020 up to 18" June 2022.

So to end with, what was everyone dying of during covid? Let's ask a death registrar what they think.

"It's the doctor's preference and his medical opinion – yet the national attention given, medical research dollars, and yearly health choices we all make are swayed by which ever cause this particular doctor, with his/her own particular training and personality, decides to jot down on the worksheet and send back to me to enter into the official record." [37]

With this in mind, remember the funding hospitals were offered for every covid death they put down and you decide what you think they will write in that 'Cause of Death' bracket. And then there are the suicide and drug overdose rates which I haven't even touched on here and yet still the death rates did not reflect a pandemic…

Finally there is also the vaccine and 5G trials which probably made a lot of people very sick in the first place making the bogus treatments also worse than useless – covered in 'Something You Should Know'.

Addendum

New article on viroliegy.com on the pollution angle which goes into more detail than in this article. [38]

---

[37] The Untrivial Pursuit
https://www.facebook.com/notes/2380732755567287/
[38] https://viroliegy.com/2022/01/28/the-covid-19-and-air-pollution-connection/

WHAT IF CANCER IS NOT A DISEASE BUT A CURE?

We all have our own personal stories of loss and pain from this dreaded so-called disease so many of you will be saying "What the hell am I on about? How did a cure kill my mum?".

My journey started with my own mum, diagnosed before the tender age of 45 with breast cancer, she followed all the doctors recommendations. She suffered horribly, not from the cancer (there is a 70+ year old Russian woman living in the back end of beyond, who's been walking around with a 20 year cancerous tumour on her breast and she is alive and well). My mum suffered from the treatments and she died one day after the 5 year survival rate of that protocol so putting her down as a success statistic. A dead success.

About 5 years ago I did a talk on Sallie O'Elkordy's radio show and have had a few requests to transcribe it. [39]

I won't put you through that but I will use it as a basis for this article.

After my mother's death at 49 I lived in fear of my own demise which mainstream media told me would be my fate as it was all down to my bad genes. I genuinely believed I would not see 50.

That changed when I had my own personal scare believing the end was nigh for me too. Finding a hard lump on my right breast I was so panicked I literally ran the half mile to my doctor's office without an appointment and grabbed the receptionist demanding to see a doctor NOW because I have breast cancer. After a brief exam I was told it was mastitis and not cancer. That was not good enough for me. I was not convinced, so in my ignorance of mammograms and the damage they do I begged to be sent for a 'proper' breast examination. At a top London cancer hospital I suffered the indignity of having my breast squeezed in a vice gladly, after which a nice doctor sat me down for a talk. He asked me why at such a young age I wanted a mammogram so I told him my history to which he replied the genetic thing is total nonsense. The media lies did not reflect the science and I had no more chance of getting breast cancer than anybody.

My mother's genes were not going to kill me.

That was the switch flipped for me. I'd been living in fear of a lie so what else was lies? I started researching. I went down many tangents and 'rabbit holes', looked at vaccines and other drugs, alternative health modalities and even common law and conspiracies. I did a lot of

---

learning. I learned how to read scientific papers while arguing with shills online over their 'science' versus my 'pseudo-science'. After 30 years I think I have cracked it and can safely say I no longer fear the 'Big C'. Not one bit. Neither should you because it is that fear which will kill you, not the cancer.

There are so many different theories about what cancer is. The conventional theory is our own cells get out of control (proliferating) and stop dying like normal cells would after a given time period. (Different body cells have differing life-spans and the natural death of a cell is called apoptosis). They carry on dividing and building, growing into new cells that also don't die.

This theory doesn't however tell us why this happens. They can't seem to explain why the cell does this, what causes it or what will stop it. Why would our cells suddenly become seemingly 'immortal'? Yes they call them immortal, look up HeLa cells. The cells from a black woman called Henrietta Lacks' cervix who they used as a human guinea pig back in the 1950's.

Her cells are still growing today in labs across the world yet her family were not paid one penny for them.

These 'immortal' cells are regarded as 'rogue' cells, the enemy in the 'war on cancer' which must be fought, battled, killed even at the expense of the whole organism (that's you by the way). Ever heard the old quote "The operation was a success but the patient died"?

This war on your own bodily cells is very short-sighted and follows the matriarchal war model without stopping to think, these are a natural process of some kind of our own cells which some might think could be a survival mechanism. After all, why would our bodies be trying to kill themselves? It's a ridiculous notion from the start. Nature always seeks balance, equilibrium and nowhere in nature will you ever see an organism fight itself.

Conventional medicine considers the tumour as the 'face' of cancer. If they can 'shrink' it, cut it out, burn it or poison it along with every other cell in your body and you manage to survive for 5 years of battle, you are chalked down as a success statistic. Just like my dead mother.

Onto alternative theories, we have the 'cancer is a fungus' theory. One Italian doctor (Simoncini) swears that opening you up and hosing your tumour down with baking soda will do the trick. [40]

If that were the case then wouldn't just cutting it out also do the

---

[40] www.cancerisafungus.com/

trick though? Fungus can survive in much harsher terrains than normal cells (and bacteria) and will feed on toxic substances. They also need no oxygen to survive (anaerobic).

Scientists have even found a way of using fungi to clean up toxic oils spills in the ocean, so if we think along those lines then fungus could indeed be playing a part in something going on in the body concerning dead cells, toxins and clean-up. But where are the immortal cells in this theory? Is this something else entirely, not truly cancer but an advanced clean-up crew? This theory ties in with the toxic overload theory where the body, for whatever reason, cannot deal with some toxins so parcels them up to protect itself from harm until such time it can be dealt with.

More on this later.

Nature does not show a propensity to attack its own organism. There is no proof anywhere that this would happen so why would we believe it of our own bodies which are perfectly designed for survival in their particular environment? Do things go wrong when the environment is compromised or has nature put things in place to help us overcome and survive possible problems? From all of nature we see proof of the latter. Therefore cancer MUST be a survival mechanism.

We also have the problem of false diagnosis and overzealous aggressive treatments. Just as they now claim measles and flu to be deadly diseases (which we all know they are not) the big cancer machine is fired up, all guns blazing at the mere smell of a cancer diagnosis, just like a war-crazed army where the enemy is your own body.

This is where the early diagnosis and awareness campaigns come in to boost the figures in the war on cancer, they can't keep filling the coffers without fresh enemies to fight so they go out on fishing expeditions to reel in more customers (fodder/fuel) for their lucrative cancer machine. By getting in younger and healthier patients who may be able to actually survive the toxic treatments they can boost their survival rates too, makes them look good. No matter that you never had cancer in the first place.

My sister died two years ago. Shortly after her death it was announced that her particular form of cancer was being declassified/downgraded to not actually a cancer at all. Proof the treatment killed her then!!

The timing of first diagnosis can have an effect on your outcome too, depending on what stage of the 'disease' you are at when it is detected. You could be in the final stage of the tumour being broken down and toxins being dealt with and so well on the road to recovery but not if they get you onto their program and start pumping you full of more toxins and killing your microbiome which is in the process of cleaning up for you.

WHAT IS A TUMOUR? (1)

Our bodies have a system to deal with poisons and toxins which modern medicine has wrongly named an 'immune system'. The germ theory we'll deal with later on but for now just go with the body's ability to clean up and expel nasty stuff which could harm us. The body uses various methods and avenues to get the stuff out and the main clean up guys are in fact bacteria (no they are not the invading enemy after all) but they only need to come into action if the body cannot immediately expel said poison. If it is inhaled the body will sneeze or cough it out, if ingested the body will eject it quickly from one end or the other (or both if you're really unfortunate). If the toxins end up in the tissues (by injection say) bacteria will proliferate there to clean up dead cells killed by the toxic load, clean up the toxins and push them out through the skin, hence poxes, rashes and pustules. If these methods don't get it out then the bacteria will go into action, this we feel as general aches, pains, fevers etc.

Most people at this point will run to the doctor and come home with antibiotics which will stop the bacteria doing their clean-up job. Although everyone takes antibiotics at some point from a doctor they are also getting into us through other ways – the water, food (particularly farmed meat which is fed massive amounts of antibiotics to fatten animals quickly) and vaccines which always contain antibiotics.

Without the bacteria/energy, the body being in stress mode, the next plan of action kicks in and the body has to partition off the harmful toxins so they cannot come in contact with healthy cells, this is called a tumour (or a cyst, even a boil depending on the stage it is noticed and the location). This lump of putrid poison if found, once it is filled and formed would be diagnosed as a benign tumour. If the body builds up enough energy and microbes to deal with the toxins and it starts breaking it down it will become inflamed and might be diagnosed as an infection or a metastasizing cancer.

Finally if diagnosed at the point when it is still filling up with toxins it will be diagnosed as a full blown cancerous tumour (growing), hence the spider looking effect of the veins transporting toxins into the partition. Still in this case those pesky immortal cells may not be present so is it really 'cancer'. I'd suggest not.

WHAT IS A TUMOUR? (2)

Now we come to the real deal which has only been answered in the last 10 years for me. It explains the crazy cancerous cell proliferation and those immortal cells, the why's the causes and the astounding outcome. German New medicine, discovered by German oncologist Dr. Hamer, describes how real cancer works and how it is not trying to kill us as modern medicine would have us believe, it is helping us to survive. If you happen to be diagnosed with this real cancer it will probably be claimed to be aggressive and deadly or stage 4.

According to the New Biology (previously German New Medicine) cancer is a biological program of tissue building to facilitate surviving a trauma of some kind. This is where the massive cell proliferation comes into play which is the hallmark of cancer and so what I would call a true cancer process.

To explain it in simple terms let's take lung cancer as a classic example. Lung cancer would be set into motion by a fright where you feel your life is threatened. You actually think you are about to die. When you are shocked what is the first thing your body does? It takes a sharp intake of breath. You go into flight or fight mode and the fuel needed is oxygen. The biological program that is switched on is to build up more lung tissue to expand the area in the lung for oxygen and carbon dioxide exchange. The switch for this is in the brainstem according to Dr. Hamer and can be clearly seen on an MRI scan forming a perfect circle (looks a bit like a target board) which will be in a different part of the brain according to which organ is being affected. (Hamer's work with these brain scans has been verified and tested by other scientists in the field. He could diagnose what organ had cancer and at what stage it was at just by looking at patients brain scans).

As a side note I wonder if these circles are being diagnosed as brain tumours too? At this point when cells are proliferating at a fast rate those 'immortal cells' will have been switched on and if you happened to be tested at this point (most won't because you'll probably feel amazing) you would undoubtedly be diagnosed with an aggressive stage 3 or 4 cancer which they will tell you will kill you within months or even weeks. That's a double whammy right there, another threat to your life plus then they will poison/radiate and even chop bits of you off/out if you go along with them.

This survival mechanism can be triggered on any organ according to the type of biological shock. Some organs will work in the opposite direction, breaking tissue down in the first phase instead of building which is sometimes the case in breast cancer which can work both ways. If a woman sadly loses a child, to deal with the shock, the milk ducts which are no longer needed and full of milk will be dismantled so the milk can be stopped and recycled to feed the body as it will be in fight or flight mode again. Once the initial shock is over and the program progresses, the milk ducts must be built back at which point the area can become 'inflamed' and may look like mastitis. (This process must be going on and on in dairy cows who regularly have bouts of mastitis and tumours as their calves are taken from them to use their milk, hence the regular doses of antibiotics. Never chemo though).

A major factor in this process is the role of bacteria. In particular tuberculin seems to be very important in the breakdown of tumours, yes the bacteria they tell us causes TB. If the specific bacteria earmarked for the job of dismantling, recycling tumours and cleaning out their contents are not present because too many antibiotics have decimated the microbiome, then what happens?

Chemo is also antibiotic except it not only kills bacteria it also kills our cells. If we look at the work of many microbiologists there is evidence that the microbes are not actually killed by antibiotics at all. They are pleomorphic, which means they can change their form to suit their environment. This is why they say 'superbugs' happen in places like hospitals. They are not superbugs, they are the same bacteria morphing to survive. If the fungal forms of our bacteria are the most durable then this might be why they are found in tumours and why Simoncini said "cancer is a fungus."

So chemo and antibiotics can impede our bacteria but not kill them. The tumour would be broken down much quicker during the final biological phase according to GNM if we refused all their drugs in other words, plus the body wouldn't have the added toxins to deal with. In short doing nothing at all is better for your outcome than any of their treatments.

So back to the other tumours that are not true cancer but are some kind of protection from toxic overload by sealing toxins off into little compartments. These also will only be broken down when the body is strong enough and can produce enough of the right microbes. If the tumour is very acidic then fungus will be present and cleaning up the toxins from the inside of the tumour, once this is done and the toxins are neutralized then the tumour can be dismantled. Then there will be a lot of bacteria on site creating heat and cell debris which modern medicine calls an infection.

So there you have it – the healing process is called a disease and must be prevented by modern medicine with their weapon of choice {drumroll} antibiotics!! Anti-life that means. The cleaning up process will not kill you, that is just ridiculous, what will kill you is the poisonous drugs that not only stop the cleaning up process but also add to the workload of new piles of toxins and debris.

I don't know if you've heard the recent fuss about measles or chickenpox in childhood lowering cancer risk in later life? I'd just like to comment on that briefly because it ties in with their false notion of germs causing disease. How can a disease on the one hand be trying to kill you yet on the other be protecting you from being killed later on? Again they contradict themselves. Firstly they have never yet managed to prove any microbe causes any disease. Secondly they have never isolated a single virus so how do you think they are going to give someone measles to cure their cancer? [41]

(Yes this is what they are purportedly trying to do and probably want to fail on purpose for obvious reasons).

It has been observed in several cases that a fever seems to send cancer into remission. Well whoop de doo!! So after what I've pointed out above WHAT do you think is happening there? The clean-up crew have arrived fully loaded. The fact that statistically kids that had measles etc. do not get cancer as adults suggests their bodies have cleaned out so no toxic build-up and also don't forget it means they were not vaccinated so lack of more toxins AND antibiotics. Their bodies are just working optimally.

So if there is no cure for a bodily clean-up or a biological process the men in white coats call 'cancer' what is the best thing to do? I am no medical doctor so am not allowed to give medical advice, so I won't, but I'd suggest you steer well clear of all of it.

Listen to your body. If you are tired, rest. Don't keep pumping yourself full of caffeine and ignoring what your body wants. Eat clean, organic species specific foods. Isn't it funny how they know exactly what to feed every animal in the zoo to keep that animal well yet they refuse to nail down the optimal human diet. Look into 'natural hygiene' and the 80-10-10 diet and why Gerson Therapy works. [42]

---

[41] www.wissenschafftplus.de/uploads/article/Dismantling-the-Virus-Theory.pdf

[42] https://innatechoice.com/downloads/The_Innate_Diet.pdf

Anyone who tells you otherwise is selling you something you don't need. If you feel nauseous or simply not hungry then fast. Fasting is the best way to rest and conserve energy for detoxing. Again listen to what your body is asking for.

Finally and most importantly you need to understand your body is trying to save you, not kill you like oncologists would have you believe. You have to let go of that fear and trust in your body. Fearing anyone in a white coat would be more appropriate than believing your body is out to get you. [43]

* There's a podcast about this on Odysee if you want to listen * [44]

---

[43] Further reading:

www.ncbi.nlm.nih.gov/pmc/articles/PMC3926122/

www.totalhealthinstitute.com/german-new-medicine/

[44] www.odysee.com/@northerntracey:a/Fakeologist-on-14-Dec-21-01-08-36_mp4_Low_:6

GOING VIRAL – A RECIPE FOR DISASTER

I touched on the invention of the virus in the chapter 'The Germ Theory – An Idiots Guide' but did not go into detail yet, so now that you've hopefully absorbed that the germ theory is wrong and contagion is also a myth I thought it might be time to delve into the virus theory, how it came about and why and to break down the wall of 'pseudo-science' they've built up around it.

The story of how viruses came about seems really complicated and 'sciencey' and that is on purpose. A bit like how they wrote the bible originally in Latin so the common people couldn't read it for themselves but had to rely on priests to deliver the message using their own agenda and their interpretations. Now they use Latin again in biological science to keep us in the dark so we have to listen to the new priests in this new cult – doctors.

There are scientists speaking out but they are still using their own language which can be daunting. So I will try and keep it as simple as I can and hopefully interesting. Once you get a look behind the curtain, see what's really been going on you won't fall for the dramatic nonsense most of the big talkers and controlled opposition are pushing.

Only recently I read a post all about the Fauci case before congress where Rand Paul questioned Fauci on his funding of something they call '**Gain of Function**'. This will hopefully show you what that actually means and why all this talk of bio-weapons is not something to freak out about per-se but more of a thing to keep an eye on because what they have done and are doing is much more ludicrous than the conspiracists say.

So to start with let's look at the beginnings, where it all started. As I said the germ theory was teetering on very shaky foundations from the start but with no internet back then it was easy to promote an idea and hush dissenters which were the scientists themselves and physicians.

From Béchamp to Rife and many doctors in between, even Florence Nightingale, all were saying germ theory couldn't work and proving it so something had to be concocted using their circular reasoning to shut them up. Something no-one could see to keep us in the dark.

The word virus pre-1930 was already being referred to as a poisonous liquid. Something no-one could see even under a microscope. Something that passed through the finest filter. Hence they called it a filterable virus/poison. Even today they claim Beijerinck discovered the first virus yet what he actually discovered was again, that germs were NOT the cause so it had to be something else and he used the word virus in the old meaning (poison). They leave out the bit about the meaning of that word at the time though.

They show pictures of this tobacco mosaic virus to this day despite it not even looking like a virus and being far too big. The pictures are in fact just pictures of a type of plant cell called a xylem cell which moves water and nutrients up and down the stem of the plant. So the picture is a fraud. How many plant scientists though link this to human biology and recognize it's not a virus because they have been compartmentalised? I spotted it straight away when I was shown it on a plant science course, but then I'm not stuck in one 'ology' box.

If you check Wikipedia's history of the virus they claim many people discovered viruses before 1931 which cannot be true because that was before the invention of the electron microscope so there was actually no proof of their claims. The only thing they WERE proving was it wasn't bacteria causing the diseases they were studying.

These 'discoveries' were all the results of taking samples of pus or sputum from sick people, filtering it and voila, they've discovered a new virus. Nothing to see here. Also none of Koch's Postulates were fulfilled with any of these new virus discoveries, they just seemed to have thrown those out the window again. They were even making vaccines from this gunk for years, just soldiering on like the blind leading the blind or was it fraud? They kept using this crude blind method to claim discovery of many supposed viruses including the ones they claimed were causing cancers like the SV40 everyone raves about. No isolation was ever done just vials of ingredients from tumours being called viruses. Strange though that cancer is not contagious yet viruses are? Anyone noticed that glaring error in their story?

Going back to 1858 Rudolf Virchow wrote his **cell theory** which said that the cell was the smallest unit of life and that the cell could produce poisons which they called 'virus' back then and that this poisonous liquid produced disease. He also said the cell was the smallest unit in biology which we know is not true. This was an hypothesis, an idea, which was never verified in science. So Beijerinck's discovery of the TMV was based on this theory AND his use of the word 'virus' meant poison. So he believed the poison was coming from the cells just like viruses today are said to do.

This virus theory (poison produced by the cells) was generally agreed on until the 1920's-30's. Then after the taking over of medical colleges by the Rockefellers and their new registration system which made only medicine based on germ theory available, they also changed the definition of the word virus in the medical dictionaries followed by the general dictionaries.

In 1935 Wendell Stanley, using a new microscope called an electron microscope, re-examined the tobacco mosaic virus and found it was mostly made of protein. In 1939, Stanley and Max Lauffer separated the virus into protein and DNA or rather RNA but that's another story. Just think genetic material. This becomes important later.

So now mixing all this together (cell theory, germ theory and what they saw under the new microscope) instead of viruses being a poison liquid produced in the cells it was changed to a pathogenic microbe (too small to see with a microscope) consisting of genetic material wrapped in protein which could invade (like germs supposedly did) and attack you from the outside-in. This despite never seeing anything attack or invade because electron microscopes can only look at dead stuff in a vacuum. Nothing living or moving.

DNA is not living or a microbe. Did you know that the double helix they say is what DNA looks like was based on a woman's X-ray photograph called Picture 51? Just like 'Area 51' her discovery was kept quiet. Rosalind Franklin worked out using this picture, chemistry reasoning and mathematics, the famous double helix (which is being challenged now so might also be wrong). So no-one has seen this DNA structure, it's all imagined again.

DNA is said to be chemicals in crystal form. Definitely NOT alive. The protein is also not living on its own as it is just a building block. It is the stuff everything living is made from. Like a piece of Lego which on its own cannot be something living but put together with lots of other building blocks it becomes something. Like chemicals and minerals are made up of atoms, living things are made up of proteins (although proteins are also made up of atoms but you get my drift).

Rivers was the first to use the term 'obligate parasite' to describe viruses. WHERE did THAT come from? But parasites are living things and these viruses were not. They were simply particles but calling them parasites helped their circular reasoning of these particles needing a living cell to replicate – in other words OUR cells. None of this was based on science, it was purely political word salad. How can crystals and building blocks suddenly become a parasite that can make baby parasites? Ridiculous but everyone bought it, because SCIENCE.

This new convoluted version of the virus held until 1951 when some

German scientists decided to do some control experiments. This is basically like a placebo where nothing is changed or added to see if the same thing happens as in the experiment with the alleged virus or poisons.

So healthy tissues were left alone to rot naturally beside the healthy tissue damaged by the supposed virus. Both tissues ('virus infected tissues' and the non-infected) produced the exact same proteins. No difference. THAT should have been the end of that theory but instead they buried the experiments in specialist journals where no-one but other scientists would see them or understand their significance. (Max Planck Instituts fur Wissenschafts Geschichte did these experiments in Germany). At the same time the newly invented electron microscope could find no difference between the infected and non-infected tissues which they still haven't seen to this day.

So far they had based virus theory on cell theory and germ theory but they were slowly mixing in a new ingredient to their soup of theories from studying Bacterio-Phages. These are a type of spore that bacteria make when their living conditions become hostile, by acidity, poisons/toxemia or a lack of oxygen etc. They liked these phages because it fitted with their original 'cells producing poisons' theory. It fitted perfectly. BUT the spores were NOT harmful and it turns out were actually the microzyma that Béchamp spoke of in his work and Naessans also discovered and named somatids.

They seemed to be the very basis of all life, a kind of multi-seed similar to a stem cell but for microbes. This is why we often hear those news stories about viruses being the basis of all life and being found in ancient ice cores yet can still come alive like a dormant seed. THIS is the somatid or microzyma. The same ones from the pleomorphism theory. Has anyone else put these two things together and realised they are the same thing? The description of these spores is some genetic material wrapped in protein but that's not what their CGI pictures look like. They have made them look like nano-bots funnily enough and not like their CGI pictures of viruses. Probably so no-one would link the two together like I just have.

Without any evidence they claimed that phages attack bacteria, rape them, impregnate their DNA so causing the bacteria to die. But the story doesn't fit the evidence AGAIN...

Only bacteria that are extremely inbred (meaning reproducing without any contact with other bacteria or microbes) turn into phages by metamorphosis. This process of morphing was being interpreted as the phages killing the bacteria but it was simply pleomorphism. The bacteria can change forms when threatened. Bacteria that are freshly plucked from their environment never change into phages, they also don't die if phages are added to them. Each species of phage always carries the same unique DNA which is the basis of their virus theory too except that they just can't make that stick either because despite the advances in genetic science they hit a wall again. No-one could isolate DNA or RNA from any tissue or bodily fluid and show it to be the right length and composition as a virus should be by their reckoning.

On June 1st 1954 along came the next first big discovery of a virus published by Prof. John Franklin Enders which gave us the theory that cells which die in the test tube after adding supposedly infected material turned into viruses (cell theory again but now mixed with the phage theory). This method would go on to be the standard method of 'growing' viruses in the lab. This death of cells was and still is called 'isolation' of the virus even though no isolation takes place in any meaning of the word.

In their mad excitement everyone ignored the obvious, that the death of the cells in the lab was not caused by a virus, but by poisoning with antibiotics, extreme starvation by withdrawing all nutrients and by adding decomposing enzymes and THIS mixture of all these noxious things is what they use to inject into our children and call vaccines. Lanka said if this soup was directly shot into a vein it would cause instant death. That wouldn't be good for business though.

Debris from the cells that die in the laboratory are still to this day used as pictures of viruses and presented as such in scientific papers. The science of virology is that simple. A bit too simple maybe so just to add more confusion and to further bury those pesky control experiments they came up with the brilliant plan of merging virology with genetics.

Genetics was the new big thing with loads of lovely funding money and viral theory being on shallow foundations – just like germ theory it was another purely political/financial move. So suddenly viruses were no longer a 'viral protein' but a dangerous gene sequence called a viral genome.

They thought they'd discovered how viruses inject their DNA with something called reverse transcriptase and so if they detected this process it meant there was what they call a retro-virus present.

The story keeps getting more convoluted, this was their new cover story to explain how dead particles replicate or zombies have babies. It's not the viruses doing it, it's an enzyme. Reverse transcriptase is what the RT in front of PCR refers to on the PCR tests. See how this is coming together nicely?

So what's an enzyme? It's a protein which acts as a chemical catalyst. What's a catalyst? It's a chemistry term, it's 'a substance that initiates or accelerates a chemical reaction'. So if we break this all down into plain English, they found an enzyme which breaks tissues and cells down (like decomposing) and they claim it is proof there is a virus around doing it but we can't see it so let's pretend chemistry can see it.

Just to touch on antibodies here as we're talking about enzymes – antibodies are also just enzymes which are said to be involved in blood clotting. It would make sense to also assume they are around when cells die and to assist in the decomposing process probably of those bits of broken DNA. They do not 'fight viruses' or germs at all and the whole immune system story is also made up nonsense.

This Reverse Transcriptase is said to happen because of a **retro virus**. Apparently it's 'retro' because it works backwards. Instead of injecting DNA it injects RNA into the host cell which makes the DNA make more RNA. But hang on, if RNA is only half a strand of DNA it could be just broken DNA from the decomposing process, right? So this is how they solved that pesky problem of not being able to find the whole viral DNA before. They just changed the story again. There is little proof that anything they've told us about DNA is even true, it's very like early virus theory with no visual proof of its existence or functions. So just like the pathogen got smaller and smaller as microscopes got better, no-one can now see what is supposedly causing disease again. We've just gone round in another circle.

I didn't want to get into DNA or retro viruses exactly because it is one of their circular arguments which sends you round and round on a never ending chase for something to make sense. After you've been around the block a couple of times you realise you always end up back where you started though. They haven't isolated any virus yet so how can any of this be based on facts let alone science? It's all just convoluted stories, laying a false trail of crumbs to keep you and I busy and not looking at the whole picture. You can get totally lost in the details. This is exactly why they have merged biology with technology to keep us continually in the dark.

It had to be done I'm afraid.

So, onwards.

In 1983 RT-PCR was invented within genetics research and was quickly pegged as the new wonder tool to spot retro viruses coz remember they've merged now. This virus test that is used is a genetic test. The genetic sequences the test seeks were never isolated from any virus as I've explained. It picks up typical bits of genetic sequences, which are released in increasing quantities when tissues and cells die. These short genetic sequences are component parts of the human metabolism, in other words it's bits of your own DNA. It picks up fragments not whole strands so they fill in the gaps with computer modelling, fill 'em in with whatever they choose. A bit like trying to do a jigsaw with missing pieces so you take some bits out of another jigsaw puzzle with missing pieces and use those bits to try and make it look like the picture on the box.

Unknown or NOVEL gene sequences or viruses cannot be found with a PCR test. First, the isolation and sequencing of a virus has to be done to develop a PCR test for it, which has to come from the virus, which they have never isolated. Round and round it goes.

This wonderful new gene lab tool became the virus industry's greatest marketing ploy. Now they could tell anyone they were infected with their own DNA!! It also became the tool they use to claim a virus isolation. Since its invention all papers claiming isolation of a new virus are done only using PCR and gene sequencing, cutting out all the problematic lab work which never found any viruses. It also resurrected the original reason the germ theory failed as a reason viruses do not, namely asymptomatic carriers. Like Typhoid Mary we are all sick we just don't know it and everyone can be a serial killer. I'm gob smacked that people even buy this crap. When they found germs in healthy people that were meant to be making them sick it threw germ theory out the window which was why they invented the virus. Yet now the same theme is being played out again so they took the opposite theory, the Terrain Theory and pleomorphism, slapped it on top and bingo – they have viruses morphing and lying dormant (like phages and bacteria again). Checkmate. Or was it?

It seems their plans for medical world domination hit another hurdle in 2016 when Stefan Lanka challenged the worlds' virologists to produce the proof of one virus. His public challenge went like this:

"The sum of 100,000 Euro will be paid on presentation of a scientific publication, in which the existence of the measles virus is not only claimed, but actually proven, and in which the diameter of the virus is determined."

Many have heard of this case which should have shattered the whole industry except they only printed half the story in the press. The half they liked. The story the world was told was that Lanka lost the bet when Bidens offered up 6 papers, the first of which was the Enders paper we already touched on earlier. The other five were just props to try and fill in the missing bits from the first paper which did not prove any viruses were found.

Of course judges can't understand the scientific papers any better than most of us can so the papers were accepted on face value and the matter had to go back to court over the none payment of the prize money. By appealing the decision Lanka got to explain the meaning of those papers and demonstrate the fraud and the false claim thereby winning the case at the appeal. There was no control experiment in any of the papers. Lanka also paid an independent lab to perform the control experiments 60+ years later and presented the results to the court. This second part of the story was totally ignored by the press. The scientists and sceptics all ganged up on the story claiming sour grapes and details were poured over but it still stands that the measles virus was not proven to exist. As I always like to point out, why would they find it so difficult to produce the proof of a virus they've been supposedly pumping into millions of kids since the 1950's?

It technically should be a walk in the park.

This second appeal case quietly happened in 2017 and I had been doing my own research and often used a website called The Big Picture Book of Viruses. [45]

I noticed in 2017 that the picture of the measles virus was taken down and the letters N/A left in their place. Not Applicable? Amazing, so glad I got a screenshot of it before they rearranged the whole site. Someone was obviously taking the verdict more seriously than they wanted to admit. Now all the fake pics are under Latin names again so none of you will bother looking at their fakery. It's only for the initiated cult members.

---

[45] www.virology.net/big_virology/bvviruslist.html

	paramyxovirus
	paramyxovirus
N/A	Measles virus
	Rinderpest virus
	Rinderpest virus

Screenshot from The Big Picture Book Of Viruses

Legally they now could be done for fraud because of that court case. Here's what was said about it by the clerk of the court…

The highest court confirmed judgement in the measles virus trial has removed the basis of the whole of virology. Not only that, it has been established in case law now that the method used since 1954 to prove viruses exist is no longer valid in 2016 and beyond. This one case should have been the end of the vaccine industry too.

Do you think this might have made them need to change the face of vaccines again? I think so. It must have.

Since this case it seems like the science of virology has gone into overdrive in pushing the fear factor of their unproven and now challenged virus theory using their usual tack of Latin word salads. For a while they stopped using the word virus and changed to proteins and phages and even prions. I noticed this change but many didn't. But now suddenly they've come back with a vengeance. Reminds me of a boxer after a bad round coming out all guns blazing. To try and hide their bruises they've plumped for total obfuscation wrapped up in computer modelling, mathematics and playing with gene fragments like a Meccano set, trying to manually build their fantasy virus genome into reality. THIS is where the 'gain of function' comes in I mentioned at the start. SO what is gain of function?

Basically it's taking something harmless which they had plumped to play the part of a virus (the Mirzoyan perhaps or maybe some protein?)

and trying to make it do what they've always told us a virus does. Trying to make it act the part of the villain. They are actually trying to make Pinocchio into a real boy in real life.

This IS the bio-weapon that all the truthers are shouting about but the mistake everyone makes is thinking they CAN do it when in reality they haven't even passed the first hurdle yet. They haven't even proved their viruses are real. They are not trying to make a dangerous super virus/bio weapon they are actually just trying to make one virus. Because in reality they haven't found one yet. It's even in plain sight with their 'protein spikes' taking the place of a virus now. Can't you see how they're muddying the waters?

But the PCR tests were a boon for finding any gene sequence they want in anyone they want to making potentially the whole world infected so looking like a contagious disease. And that's exactly what they did. What these tests are actually picking up is bits of our own microbiome's DNA fragments (also from our own bacteria, remember those phages). Bacteria have much more DNA than our own cells so these so-called variants and mutations could keep going forever unless we all know the game they're playing. Also it is now well known that our DNA does change, is not fixed at all. Epigenetics is well known now thanks to Bruce Lipton. This is how Lanka explains these 'mutations' – here comes a bit of science...

Sequence alignment is a bioinformatics technique in which fragments of nucleic acid (DNA) are assembled with a computer into a hypothetical strand of genetic material. In order to carry out the alignment, roughly comparable to a jigsaw puzzle, templates in the form of old strands of genetic material are required. In the same way as the picture on the box of a puzzle serves as a template. In the case of SARS-CoV-2, two old corona models were used for this purpose.

Because during the alignment process, large parts of the constructed genome strand are invented, and other parts are 'tweaked' by the associated computer programs to produce a reasonably credible result, the finished product never looks 100% like the template. It's similar to forcibly putting together puzzle pieces that don't even belong to the original to create a similar image and voila, new variant.

To bring you up to date with this whole covid thing and the bat story and the 'escaped from a lab secret bio-weapon thing', can you work out what went on now from what I've told you in plain English? No they hadn't managed to make a virus but they did need something quick to cover up for all the vaccine deaths happening in Wuhan so they coddled together an 'in silico virus'. That is a made-up-by-a-computer virus. They took some of their SARS sequences and added some extra bits lumped together from the gene-bank where they've been storing all their genetic sequences and claimed that was the novel virus genome. Truthers found out about the gene sequences being already on the gene bank, with patents too.

The Chinese were working on several SARS/Cov vaccines and have lodged 3 SARS/COV genetic sequences with the online gene bank. They are named SARS/Cov 1, 2 and 3. All the genetic sequences were manufactured using CRISPR which means they take bits of genes from animals and humans and splice them together.

Remember, you can't patent anything from nature hence the sequences used were put together by men's hands or rather by computers and so the conspiracy theorists put 2 and 2 together to make 5. A big Chinese conspiracy which only added more fuel to the fire creating even more fear of viruses. Those truthers shouting about deadly bio-weapons and deflecting the argument to who did it only serve to boost the sales of the covid vaccines which actually were not brand new at all.

China's Mandatory Vaccination Law Went Into Effect on December 1, 2019 – The Coronavirus Outbreak is a Vaccine Experiment Gone Bad

February 19, 2020 by IWB

Screenshot of news page Investmentwatchblog.com

The fact that we are being told the vaccines for covid were rushed through is a lie. They've been working on them for almost 20 years (with no success). This was probably a human trial gone wrong of these SARS vaccines which has exploded into a worldwide trial for a totally new genetic modification of our genes which they are calling vaccines (that is fraud). They've been working on this gene therapy since the 1990's. Did they see an opportunity to silently dismantle the struggling vaccine industry and replace it with gene therapy?

They've always complained vaccines were not a big profit maker in themselves mostly because of the time it takes to make them and put them through the testing procedures which takes years but also the lack of virus proof and the anti-vax movement. Vaccines were not working and the cat was almost fully out of the bag so why carry on flogging a dead horse when big tech can come in and save the day and resurrect the dead horse into something much more lucrative? What could possibly go wrong?

Speaking of resurrecting, how about this – in 1840 inoculation was banned because it was causing smallpox. (Remember what I said about inoculations spreading across Europe seeming to cause plagues?). That's when Jenner came along did a little name swap, renaming Inoculation to Vaccination even though it's still basically the same process. Jenner was no physician, in fact in his day he would have been called a quack. He bought his doctorate papers. Jenner was a freemason by the way.

You may think the timeline doesn't fit this name swap as the ban came out after his new invention, not new or invented, unless you know how long these new laws take to be implemented. Freemasons are always in the thick of politics and medicine so was this a pre-empting of the coming ban? Looks like it to me. Looks like more political dirty dealing for big profits.

Always use Occums Razor when dealing with their stories, meaning always look for the simplest explanation because the truth is always simple. Lies are convoluted and go round in circles, hence the mutations and variants and the ever changing story of what viruses are. So rather than fearing these mad scientists we should be locking them up, they really are deluded.

Instead of laughing at conspiracy nuts who shout 'no virus isolation' go and see if what I've said here is true. Look at the methods used. They are always what I've told you here. Read Stefan Lanka's papers which are challenging not only the whole of virology but the whole medical system too. His latest challenge is out there now, it's called Projekt Immanuel.

He has challenged the worlds virologists to do the control experiments never done since 1951 for Covid-19. He has already done them himself, it's now up to the rest of them to put up or shut up. If viruses were real they should have NO problem with this. The problem is though, is anyone going to listen? Remember the same people own the media that own medicine and big celebrities and top politicians. You will not hear anything about this from any of them.

Like George Carlin said "It's one big club and YOU ain't in it."

WORDS, MEANINGS, MONEY AND POWER

Words and their meanings can be changed organically over time (a long time) but someone has been manipulating words for personal monetary gains for the last century at least.

Gay used to mean happy, jolly, colourful in days gone by. It was adopted by the homosexual community but strangely not so much the lesbians. Not sure why they always say 'gay and lesbian' and why lesbians can't be included in the happy, jolly community? Recently it has been usurped again to be used as a 'diss' as in 'that's so gay' meaning lame, stupid. This process seems to have been quite organic unless someone knows otherwise.

The bible was probably the first use of word manipulation when it was finally translated from Latin for the common people. The word 'MEAT' is a clear example of smoke and mirrors. Meat in biblical terms means FOOD. It does not mean the flesh of a dead animal. This was not re-translated in most versions because Constantine who had a hand in the writing of it didn't think people would convert to Christianity if they knew the early Christians were vegetarians. They covered that up to make the religion more popular.

Christianity and religion WERE politics originally used in the power structure. A 'vegan' leader would not be good for numbers though.

More recently we've seen the changing of some of the 'medical' definitions in everyday dictionaries and how they can change the political landscape.

In the 1930's when the Rockefellers were taking over the 'healing practices' and turning everything towards chemical based allopathy, the word VIRUS was redefined in all the dictionaries by these chemical/oil barons. Why?

Because Virus used to mean 'poison' or 'venom'. Chemicals ARE mostly poisonous (at least the ones produced by the oil industry as a sideline to become big pHarma).

The word pharmacy is also an interesting word if you find the original meaning of it. Pharmacy is derived from the Greek word pharmakeia, meaning 'use of drugs, medicines, potions, or spells; poisoning, witchcraft; remedy, cure' AND the Bible reveals that Babylon will deceive all nations by the use of pharmacy that is in connection to 'magical arts and idolatry'.

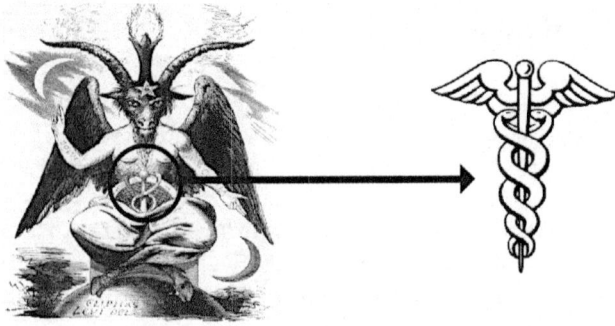

There's an interesting article about the word and what's hidden behind it on the 'Assembly of Called-Out Believers' website. [46]

Back to the dictionary and the word Virus…

> **virus | Origin and meaning of virus by Online Etymology …**
> https://www.etymonline.com/word/virus
>
> **virus** (n.) late 14c., "poisonous substance" (a sense now archaic), from Latin **virus** "**poison**, sap of plants, slimy liquid, a potent juice," from Proto-Italic *weis-o-(s-) "**poison**," which is probably from a PIE root *ueis-, perhaps originally meaning "to melt away, to flow," used of foul or malodorous fluids, but with specialization in some languages to "poisonous fluid" (source also of Sanskrit visam "venom, **poison**," visah "poisonous;" Avestan vish-"poison;" Latin viscum "sticky substance …

Now some may say it changed because 'science' evolved but that would be what they want you to think. No, it changed because of money, greed and power. Besides, at the time of the change no-one had yet SEEN this new redefined virus at all.

So science was not behind the change but maybe 'science' as in the bought kind was.

Here are the more recent definitions before covid:

A: The causative agent of an infectious disease.

B: Any of a large group of submicroscopic infective agents that are regarded either as extremely simple microorganisms or as extremely complex molecules, that typically contain a protein coat surrounding an RNA or DNA core of genetic material but no semipermeable membrane, that are capable of growth and multiplication only in living cells, and that cause various important diseases in humans, lower animals, or plants; also, filterable virus.

C: A disease or illness caused by a virus.

---

[46] www.calledoutbelievers.org/pharmakeia-and-bio-pharma/

In 2014 they were still saying this:

vi·rus 🔊 *noun* \'vī-rəs\

: an extremely small living thing that causes a disease and that spreads from one person or animal to another

: a disease or illness caused by a virus : a viral disease

So still a kind of 'germ' not too long ago. (Page captured from Merriam-Webster dictionary in August 2014, Waybackmachine).

This clearly shows they were using 'viruses' to prop up the germ theory as microscopes proved the germs were not the cause of any disease.

Had to include this Google remnant which seems to have been forgotten.

Virus definition and meaning | Collins English Dictionary
https://www.collinsdictionary.com/dictionary/english/virus
Virus definition: A **virus** is a kind of germ that can cause disease. | Meaning, pronunciation, translations and examples

Now during the covid plandemic they have gone after the dictionary definition of 'VACCINATION'. You might have heard people decrying these new shots are NOT vaccines but why does it matter? Well again, greed, money and this time so much more.

Here is the recent definition of vaccination, again from Merriam-Websters for continuity:

vaccine noun

vac·cine | \ vak-'sēn 🔊, 'vak-ˌsēn\

Definition of *vaccine*

: a preparation of killed microorganisms, living attenuated organisms, or living fully virulent organisms that is administered to produce or artificially increase immunity to a particular disease

So 'micro-organism' means bacteria/germs NOT viruses.

I might point out that the original word came from Vacca, meaning cow, because Jenner used the pus from cows with cowpox to inoculate against smallpox. Inoculations were about to be banned so he coined the name vaccination to get round the ban and giving all the use of the process to only registered medics. Money and power again. This definition is describing 'inoculation' which was banned in the late

1800's. I suppose they think everyone has forgotten about that and I suppose they would be right.

Using the Waybackmachine again:

We can see that in January of 2021 right when the covid shots were being rolled out, this happened to the dictionary definition of a vaccine.

vaccine noun

🔖 Save Word

vac·cine | \ vak-ˈsēn 🔊, ˈvak-ˌsēn \

Definition of *vaccine*

: a preparation that is administered (as by injection) to stimulate the body's immune response against a specific infectious disease:

a : an antigenic preparation of a typically inactivated or attenuated (see ATTENUATED sense 2) pathogenic agent (such as a bacterium or virus) or one of its components or products (such as a protein or toxin)

b : a preparation of genetic material (such as a strand of synthesized messenger RNA) that is used by the cells of the body to produce an antigenic substance (such as a fragment of virus spike protein)

WOW that is some big difference overnight particularly part B. How convenient to make gene 'therapy' magically sit under the umbrella of vaccines so they can get emergency authorization to test their gene modification on all humans on the planet. That is some feat of word definition manipulation for money, greed and power right there. It's under your noses.

Again some will argue that it has changed to 'catch up' with 'science'. If that was really the case it would not be pre-empting the results of this 'vaccine/gene manipulation' TRIAL. It is a trial. The results will not be in until 2023 (as of today we're still waiting) therefore it has not been scientifically verified to be a successful or verified scientific experiment. To top that off they have openly stated the shots 'do not provide immunity' nor do they claim to 'prevent transmission' both of which still mean they cannot be claimed to be 'vaccines'. Now this means the shots and the changed definitions in the dictionaries are tantamount to FRAUD.

Now do you see why word definitions are so important and how they can be manipulated for political and monetary gains?

Personally I see this as desecration of dictionaries and words. It shouldn't be allowed. In this particular case clearly a crime is being committed on several fronts.

"And the light of a candle shall shine no more at all in thee; and the voice of the bridegroom and of the bride shall be heard

no more at all in thee: for thy merchants were the great men of the earth; for by thy sorceries were all nations deceived."
– Revelation 18:23

We certainly ARE being deceived but by whom and why?

Follow the money…

The importance of meanings of words should not be diminished or changed for profit. Someone left this comment on my article 'Ex-Spurts-Who Do You Listen To?' which I feel is relevant here.

"A video by Max Igan I've just watched suggests words are a spell. I tend to agree. I speak more than one language and am a "qualified" teacher of English. The word "qualification", in language, means to define meaning more precisely. For example an adjective "qualifies" a noun. The adjective "red" qualifies the noun "car." The qualification also limits. The red car is taken away from cars in general. So, we often ask whether a person "is qualified to comment", as if this gives the qualified person a particular power. No, what it really does is indicate that person's limitation (in terms of their qualification). Seen in this light, qualifications are limitations and not anything to hold in awe. In my personal life I have found this to be true." Thanks Ian.

Dictionary definitions are used in matters of law and crimes. Can words be changed in law dictionaries? I don't think so. They can be added to but not taken away from. Words have power and should be used wisely. Like this from Authority Pub. [47]

7 Tips for Making Your Written and Spoken **Words** Powerful
  1. Speak the truth.
  2. Avoid exaggerations.
  3. Don't use double standards.
  4. Don't use your **words** to manipulate others.
  5. Be consistent in what you say.
  6. Speak mindfully.
  7. Use **words** to benefit others.

All these 'rules' have been broken now.

On words as 'spells' the clue is in the word.

The first thing you learn when you go to school is how to spell.

Words are *spells* to create a **sentence** of **terms**. [48]

---

[47] https://authority.pub › power-of-words
[48] www.dtss.us/blog/words-are-spells/

The changing of these definitions is a crime and if it isn't then dictionaries just lost their authority over the meanings of words for us all.

I was sent a video of Jordan Grant after writing this and he said something very pertinent which I'd like to add here, so I snipped this bit out of his talk, the entirety of which is well worth a listen to. [49]

> When you are writing laws you are testing words to find their utmost power. Like spells, they have to make things happen in the real world, and like spells, they only work if people believe in them.
>
> Hilary Mantel

Proteins, Spikes and Bio-weapons

All this talk of spike proteins and no-one knows what they are actually talking about. [50]

For years we've had an obsession with protein in the diet. "Where do you get your protein from?" is a question constantly asked of plant-based eaters. The question clearly shows the asker does not understand what proteins are. In the case of diet we do not get protein from eating 'protein'. Our body MAKES proteins from amino-acids. If you eat complex proteins that are already formed, the body has to dismantle or unfold the protein to extract the amino-acids which it needs to build its own proteins. This process of breaking down takes a lot of energy and creates 'acids' which have to be buffered to keep the body PH more alkaline.

Calcium is the buffer. If you get acid reflux what neutralizes that? Rennie's. What's the main ingredient of Rennie's? Chalk. What's chalk? Calcium. So to digest protein the body uses up a lot of calcium. Hence the increase in osteoporosis on the high protein western diet. Where can we get the original building blocks (amino-acids) from to cut out this wasteful process? Raw fruits and vegetables. (Cooking destroys a lot of amino-acids).

Our cells make many different shapes of protein – just like Lego pieces, there are different ones for different uses. Some are building blocks for making tissues/cells, all manner of things that make up the physical body. There are proteins that work as enzymes or solvents; basically there are lots of different combinations of amino-acids to form lots of different types of proteins so the amino-acids are the building blocks of proteins. All this info is from traditional scientific teaching. Right or wrong it is what we are going to work with because it is what THEY are working with.

So far we've just dealt with protein in the digestive system which technically is not 'inside' the body proper. Think of the body like a donut and the digestive tract is the hole in the middle of the donut, there is a tissue barrier between the digestive tract and the rest of the body so whole proteins will not end up in the blood or the nervous system or the rest of the body tissues. Why is this important? You'll soon find out. (Keep leaky gut in mind though).

---

[50] Listen to the podcast here:
www.bitchute.com/video/bLAerhc96IJD/

An example is when you put your finger in the hole of a doughnut. Your finger is NOT in the doughnut. If you **imagine your G.I. tract as an elongated doughnut**, then you can see the similarity.

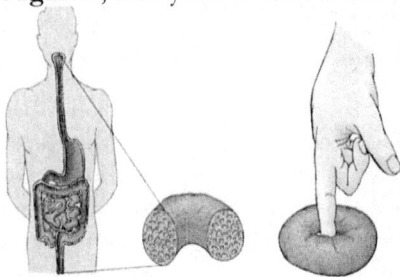

In 1903 a scientist called Nicholas Maurice Arthus was busy poisoning rabbits with various 'protein poisons' and venoms. He was trying to work out how 'immunity' happened, the process Pasteur had theorized in his germ theory and people had been trying to produce with their home-made inoculations. Arthus though was working with poisons (poison proteins) and venoms. He discovered the 'Arthus Reaction'.

This is where it gets interesting because he discovered that injection of a protein didn't cause a reaction the first time BUT if injected again with the same protein the poor animals would suffer as if they had been severely poisoned. Kind of killing the whole inoculation theory of 'immunity' which had been based on tolerance build up to chemical poisons, like alcohol for instance.

In 1905 Rossenau and Anderson (yes – the same ones who did the famous failed contagion experiments) discovered this same process but this time found the reaction happened with ANY proteins (not just poison proteins) using things like cow's milk, serum, eggs and muscle extract. They also noted that the dose did not matter, the tiniest dose would still cause a huge reaction.

This reaction was called ANAPHYLAXIS.

In 1907 another scientist called Richet, working on the same thing but this time on poor dogs, found that if you took the blood from an animal that had been 'anaphylaxised' (they had had the 1st injection and were primed for the reaction now) and injected it into a healthy animal they would have an anaphylactic reaction straight away despite not being 'primed'. Did this mean the animals chemistry had been changed making its own blood poisonous?

This was never answered.

(Is this why they don't want blood from 'vaccinated' people now in blood banks?).

He also worked out that there was an incubation period between the 1st injection and the 2nd one producing the horrific anaphylactic effect. It had to be at least 2 weeks (3-4 weeks was the average) for anaphylaxis to occur on a 2nd injection. Once primed and the 2nd injection given the result would be total shut down of the nervous system.

Richet went on to receive a Nobel prize for this 'momentous discovery' which makes one wonder how the vaccine industry can flat out lie and tell us vaccines do not cause allergies.

Are there proteins in vaccines? Yes of course, lots of them and some are common foodstuffs which they don't have to list in the ingredients as they are considered GRAS despite knowing the anaphylaxis process!!! One of the famously unlisted proteins they used in vaccines was PEANUT OIL. Are you starting to join the dots yet?

Just like they kept changing the names of diseases to hide vaccine failures they now seem to be calling anaphylaxis by new names too. Cytokine storm. ADE (Antibody Dependent Enhancement).

Now we should look at their fairytale description of a 'virus' again. 'Some genetic material wrapped in a PROTEIN shell.' Hmm. Could this have been a convenient lie to accommodate their having to inject foreign proteins into our children or just a coincidence?

We've known since 2017 that they have no viruses and they've been using various words to negate this like bacteriophage, antigen, viral genes/particles, prions and PROTEIN. But suddenly in 2020 they were not only proudly shouting about viruses again, they've added PROTEIN SPIKES into the mix.

Is this like a magic, sleight of hand trick they're pulling or are they just seriously confused by their own convoluted lies now?

WHY do you think they are so obsessed with pumping us full of proteins? Proteins are not viruses but we know now they can be used as bio-weapons and have been for many years in vaccines. They can be man-made in a lab and injected into willing subjects BUT they cannot fly around and land on you and make you sick. Just like a snake cannot spit on you and cause you to be poisoned. Not even their 'gain of function' experiments will make proteins into flying bio-weapons. They HAVE to be INJECTED, just like snake venom. But what if they are trying to induce anaphylaxis?

Look at how sensitized some children can be to peanuts. They can have a reaction simply from being close to someone eating peanuts.

Now do I have your attention? All this talk of shedding only makes sense if you have been primed to react to whatever proteins someone might be shedding. IF the shedding is even occurring. Either way, if you haven't been primed you will not react.

The 'released from a bio-lab' story is ONLY a psyop to induce more fear, to convince us that their viruses are REAL even if they are not natural.

The only truth in this story is that the 'genome' they say is from a novel virus WAS made in a lab. A gene lab. On a computer. It is a manmade gene sequence that cannot do anything because it doesn't exist except in a computer. This big lie is a cover-up for the other big lie. They have no viruses.

The fact that the mainstream media are now running this story and Facebook have taken it off their banned list speaks volumes.

The vaccines are not selling well. Not enough people are willing to risk their lives for what they see as another flu. The fear factor needed ramping up another notch. THAT is the only reason they have pulled this joker card. It's a very risky move because it could expose the WHOLE lie and they're obviously willing to take that risk to get whatever it is they want to inject into us, into us.

The prime objective is the shots, anything else will be put down to collateral.

THE AMINO AGE AND THE NEW ABNORMAL DOCTORS

MRNA is apparently the only new cure for all our ills. They're even giving this new era in medicine a name calling it the 'Amino Age' but is it all it's cracked up to be? I just heard too that 'anti-vaxxers' are trendy now which tells me they are ready to complete their big swap of vaccines for gene therapy. Problem, reaction, solution in full swing. The amino age is the offered solution but is it a solution at all or just another terrible 'healthcare' paradigm to keep the slaves manageable and controlled?

Are you confused by all this talk of 'messenger' 'RNA', proteins, genes, genomes, DNA and contagious disease? Well you're not alone and you are being confused on purpose. The way out of the confusion I thought was to dive in, swim around and see what I can find that is solid and factual in all this science-waffle being foisted on us. People with bits of paper to say they are qualified to tell us the facts are either lying or also confused.

I spent three weeks looking into their papers and articles, methods and tests and gave myself a massive headache. It reminded me of the days when I was trying to argue with shills over vaccines and what they did and did not which actually taught me a lot about their so-called science and how they confused people with their fancy language there too. All the technical stuff I learned about back then is just being rehashed and plonked onto what we are told about RNA and DNA. Just swap the word virus for DNA/RNA and you will see the same exaggerations, assumptions and lies.

I have to hit you with some big misconceptions which pull the rug from under the feet of modern medicine. This is a bit scary for some people but I promise you the truth is far prettier than the convoluted ugly theories we've been sold.

First bombshell incoming...

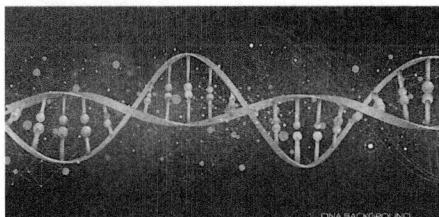

DNA. Does it exist like the pretty pictures say it does? The theory of a blueprint in the nucleus of every cell. As I was trying to knit all this info into some sort of semblance of cohesion I suddenly wondered where were the chromosomes in all this? No-one mentions them or what THEY are. SO, I looked them up.

Supposedly DNA is wrapped up in the 'chromosomes' in the nucleus of our cells which have only ever been seen when cells are dividing (only seen in embryotic cells in other words). They see these chromosomes double and split into the new cells as it divides into two. This process is called mitosis. DNA cannot be seen though, and the very few 'photo's' of what we are told is DNA are very dodgy. Two I looked for have even been deleted from the internet but I found them on the Waybackmachine.

Why did they delete them? Probably because they look so fake! Also sadly for them they look nothing like their cartoon DNA.

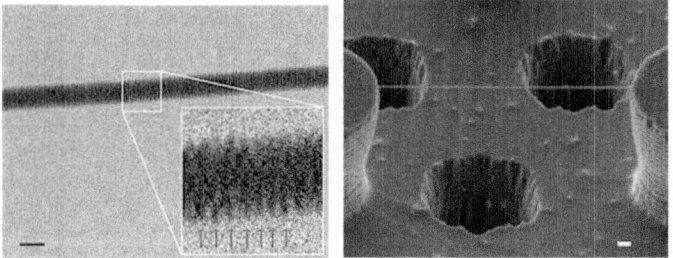

Let's see what Lanka had to say about DNA and RNA back in the 1990's (from Mark Gabrish Conlan's interview with Stefan Lanka in December 1998 issue of Zenger's Magazine).

"I already had a somewhat critical attitude when I started studying molecular genetics, so I went to the library to look up the literature on HIV. To my big surprise I found that when they are speaking about HIV they are not speaking about a virus, they are speaking about cellular characteristics and activities of cells under very special conditions. I was wondering what viruses are for in evolution because they didn't seem to have any function other than to be very dangerous and killing other cells. So I went into evolutionary biology and found that the first genetic molecule of life was RNA, and only later in evolution did DNA come into existence. Every one of our genomes, and that of higher plants and animals is the product of so-called reverse

transcription: **RNA transcribed into DNA. But I had already realized by then that the thinking about molecular genetics was very dogmatic. In the early 1960's they came up with the central dogma of molecular genetics, which they try to uphold even today, and which is ridiculous.**

The dogma says that DNA behaves in a static way (it doesn't change); DNA makes RNA; RNA cannot be transcribed back into DNA; RNA comes into existence only on the basis of DNA. That was and is the basis of the central dogma of molecular genetics. While studying the evolutionary aspects of biology, I quickly realized that reverse transcription is common to all forms of life , and in fact is the basis of all higher living. Later I learned that reverse transcription is a repair mechanism for chromosomal DNA. But the mainstream of molecular genetics is still committed to the central dogma 'there is no such thing as reverse transcription from RNA to DNA.' In 1970, when they detected biochemically that there is a reverse flow of genetic material, they didn't give up the dogma or even try to change it. Instead they called it an exception to the central dogma of molecular genetics, and explained it by postulating the existence of retroviruses"

We are told that our chromosomes (the genome) were 'mapped' by a man called Morgan but all I can find is work on plants and insects. How did he map the human chromosomes by looking at plants and insects? They used 'classical genetics' as in looking at natural mutations like Mendell (a Botanist) did with his peas which all this stuff is based on. Peas with different colored flowers. Inbreeding and cross breeding.

Chromosomes are like your sock drawer for keeping all those '6 feet' of strings of DNA in some kind of order. But it's not just one string of DNA because we have 23 paired chromosomes making 46 in all. So that's a lot of blueprints not just one.

Oh and guess what! We can SEE chromosomes under a normal microscope BUT what they are and do is something else because they are only ever seen during cells dividing, as in fetal cells. If that's the case there's no proof they are in all cells and Harold Hillman disputed this.

More recently new pics are emerging saying they don't look anything like the pictures we've been sold again. The strands of DNA are supposed to be wrapped up in a globular mess somehow? Looks like they've been looking at bacterial chromosomes (or is it just more debris?) and now they're fighting over which ones are the real deal. [51]

The new cartoon drawing of a chromosome looks just like a picture of their proteins. Like a lump of badly tangled wool. I can't help but say too, even though I might get blasted for it, that the original chromosomes look an awful lot like 'bacteria'. There I said it.

Then I remembered this from an old article I edited by Lee Stevenson, a fellow independent researcher, called 'Is It Time To Give Up On The Flawed Modern Day Science Of Genetics?'.

"They will not consider the fact that humans/animals and plants have microbes that modulate their genes. Changes in the functions of those genes also change animal and plant microbial makeup. Microbiota can alter host gene expression. These things have definitely not been considered by the biotech industry or the pharmaceutical industry. Something as simple as altering our diet can change our microbiome and alter gene expression in the body."

So are the 'genes' (small strings of protein making recipes) really coming from our own cells or are they from our bacteria? Do our cells make the proteins from reading instructions from our own 'blueprint DNA' or do the bacteria deliver them? Seeing as there is no proof whatsoever of our own cells doing this and the fact they are using bacteria and yeast to produce synthetic proteins it looks like it's all a lie, a mistake or assumptions?

All the work I looked at about producing 'synthetic RNA/DNA' seems to use bacteria and yeast to produce the product (which by the way a company called Trilink who produce it call it (RNA) a 'drug'. Funny description for something which is supposed to control our whole existence and heredity.

On the production end I just saw mixing of chemicals (acids and catalysts) with yeast and bacteria and then the usual poisoning and centrifuging plus heating and cooling till the end product pellets called 'synthetic RNA' is left and they call it a DRUG. This is what they call BIO-CHEMISTRY. Is it producing chemicals from biological processes or is it condensing living biology down to chemical processes or a bit of both? Just as they did with herbal medicines (plants) to turn them into patentable drugs.

Just for clarification we need to look up some of the things they talk

---

[51] https://3c1703fe8d.site.internapcdn.net/newman/csz/news/800/2013/xshapenottru.png

about in these 'gene modification processes'. RNA is said to be just strings of ACIDS. In their CGI illustrations they look like half a string of DNA. How do they know it has a function and how can it pass messages if it is just a string of chemicals (acids)?

What are Acids?

From the Free Dictionary: **(Chemistry) chem**

Of, derived from, or containing acid: *an acid radical.*

Being or having the properties of an acid: *sodium bicarbonate is an acid salt.*

Bicarb is supposed to alkalize so why is it classed as an 'acid salt'?

From the Cambridge Dictionary:

Acid *noun* (Chemical)

Any of various usually liquid substances that can react with and sometimes dissolve other materials.

So an acid is a 'reactive' substance, not necessarily negative. Sounds like what an enzyme does too. So in this context acids don't mean 'acids' as in acid/alkaline ok.

So what is an Amino Acid?

From the Cambridge Dictionary: **Amino Acid**

Noun **(C) Biology, Chemistry specialized**

Any of the chemical substances found in plants and animals that combine to make protein (= a substance necessary for the body to grow).

ANY chemical substance found in living tissues then.

But now look what it says about protein too.

From the Cambridge Dictionary: **Protein**

Any of a large group of chemicals that are a necessary part of the cells of all living things.

So proteins are just a mixture of chemicals too? Well in their eyes they are. So the supposed 'spike protein' is a bunch of chemicals mixed in a certain way according to them. Sounds just like a drug doesn't it? Now maybe we can understand how they might seem to make them in a chemistry lab.

There are so many scare stories coming out left right and centre about how much damage this 'spike' protein could cause, and not only to those who take the shots but maybe even those close to them who haven't, so raking up the old contagion myth once again.

We know viruses are a lie based on germ theory (another lie) but now we are made to believe proteins can suddenly spread disease person to person by 'shedding' of a fictional protein which they say they can force our own cells to produce at their bidding.

But can they?

They are mixing chemistry and mathematics and applying them to biological functions. This is the materialistic world these scientists live in. We are just breathing/walking chemical labs. We need to look at how the science of genetics has evolved seeing as it is becoming the new dominant 'science' in medicine. They brag about it replacing chemo and vaccines – well could it be any worse than chemo?

Could it be any worse than vaccines? Or is it just the same stuff repackaged with more bells and lights?

The processes in the lab look like smoke and mirrors to me all to hide the fact they either do not know what they are doing apart from chemical mixing or they do know what they are doing but don't want us to know, in fact it looks like the alchemy of old which was also very secretive and the old 'science' of the freemasons.

Let's have a look at the evolution of the smoke and mirrors.

Classical genetics was a very slow process of damaging/poisoning and observing reactions (mutations) and earlier just inbreeding. Classical genetics looked for new mutations in plants (peas originally) and fruit flies because they reproduce very quickly. When they saw a 'mutation' they blamed the genes. Genetics was all about inheriting traits but it has morphed into genes causing changes in real time. Just like they blamed germs and then viruses as scapegoats for chemical poisoning or malnutrition, they have gone now to molecular levels of invisibility.

So a plant grows with unusual features and instead of asking what caused it to grow like that they claim the reaction as the cause again. As with the TMV (Tobacco Mosaic Virus) they assumed it was something smaller than a germ (so a virus) when it was soil depletion (malnutrition). Just as pleomorphism happens and bacteria morph to survive a hostile terrain the morphism is not the cause it is a symptom. The terrain is bad. Everything has to adapt to its environment or perish.

In the 1990's they went from classical genetics to technology and invented the 'Microarrays'. Basically they take the cell debris and put each bit robotically onto a chip arranged like thousands of jigsaw pieces just like you would spread them out to see before you start doing the jigsaw except they claim to know what each bit of cell debris is and where it is placed.

Like this …

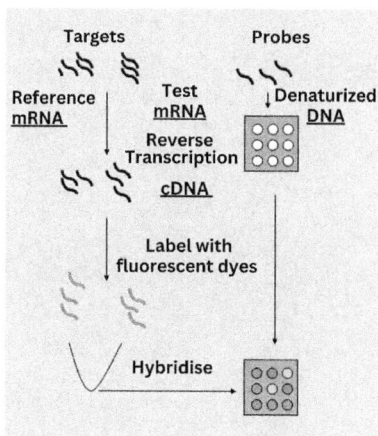

All very nice but the reactions they claim are from specific genes were identified by classical genetics using observations of reactions to terrain anomalies and lots of guesswork. Now the assumptions made have become coloured dots produced by computers, robots and chemical reactions all programmed into computers from their old poisonings, observations and guesswork. These assays were adopted from gene labs into virology labs since they announced that viruses were bits of genetic material so we can see how the two sciences were already crossing over.

All the CGI pictures of DNA and talk of 'snipping' and editing makes it sound very high tech and mysterious but do you know what they use to 'snip' and 'join' these supposed strings of acids? Bacteria.

Yeh. Apparently E-coli is a favourite 'tool' for snipping at amino-acid strings they call RNA. The same bacteria that dismantle proteins and dead tissues in our guts and also claim are very pathogenic (cause sickness). More proof that bacteria are indeed the janitors in the body and they know it. In fact it exposes they might be even more than just janitors doesn't it?

What else do they say about RNA? According to dictionary definitions it is a 'polymer'. It is some 'monomers' clumped together. Monomers are another 'chemical compound' which may or may not react with others. Plastic is a polymer, so is paper. All the info you find about these polymers and 'reactions' between proteins and acids when you look them up separately are chemical and atomic reactions. Like this from the Encyclopedia Britannica:

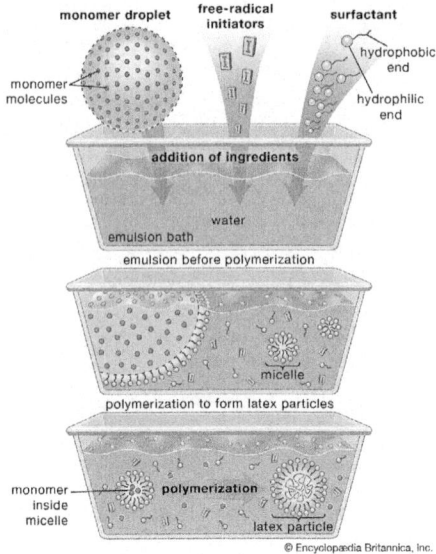

monomer droplet · free-radical initiators · surfactant

monomer molecules

hydrophobic end

hydrophilic end

addition of ingredients

water

emulsion bath

emulsion before polymerization

micelle

polymerization to form latex particles

monomer inside micelle · polymerization · latex particle

© Encyclopædia Britannica, Inc.

It is a picture of a chemical reaction yet it also looks eerily like what they claim goes on at molecular level in the body. This is chemistry overlaid onto biology. That 'polymer' looks exactly like their description of a virus doesn't it? Coincidence or plagiarism? A bit like saying all birds are aeroplanes because we can understand how aeroplanes work. We are supposed to believe the inside of our cells looks like a plastic factory in other words. So let's have a little look at how they claim to do all this gene editing and splicing which looks so high tech and clever in their cartoon pictures......

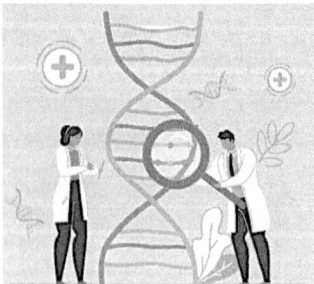

What is CAS9?

CAS9 is the protein at the heart of the CRISPR system.

CAS9 is able to take on a gRNA (guide RNA) and remove any genes that match this gRNA from the subject's DNA.

Originally, this protein was a part of bacterial immune systems.

Now it has harnessed to be an efficient and accurate tool in the world of genome editing.

What is CRISPR-CAS9?

CRISPR-CAS9 is a trailblazing genome editing tool developed by Jennifer Doudna, Emmanuelle Charpentier, and their team.

They are claiming this CAS9 is a protein from a bacteria's 'immune system'. Now that is interesting isn't it? They claim that bacteria produce proteins based on past experience of damaging chemicals just like the story of our own 'immune systems' do. So who is driving this 'immune system', is it our cells or our bacteria? Could it be that bacteria are not only our janitors but they are also our 'immune system' instead of being the enemy that our immune system was said to attack. This little nugget just tells us that THEY KNEW all along bacteria were helpers and not enemies. They clean up and they recycle cell fragments and they are trying to harness that. Problem is they only do this in our body with dead cells and debris, they do not harm or damage healthy living cells.

Remember RNA/DNA is not a living substance just like viruses were not. Are they trying to make this protein work for them on live tissue cells using 'gain of function'? There's been a big hoo-ha about 'Gain of Function' experiments and we are led to believe they have been trying to make a virus. But what about this? No mention of viruses here. Gain-Of-Function Mutations Provide Clues To The Role Genes Play In A Cell Or Organism. [52]

In the same way that cells can be engineered to express a dominant negative version of a protein, resulting in a loss-of-function phenotype, they can also be engineered to display a novel phenotype through a gain-of-function mutation. Such mutations may confer a novel activity on a particular protein, or they may cause a protein with normal activity to be expressed at an inappropriate time or in the wrong tissue in an animal. Regardless of the mechanism, gain-of-function mutations can produce a new phenotype in a cell, tissue, or organism. [53]

Is the Gain of Function story a bending of the truth (hidden in plain sight)? Are they trying to make these proteins edit genes in live cells in live subjects – US? Trying to genetically modify us under the guise of curing something. Remember what Lanka said about reverse transcription. There are lots of indications to tell us they have been failing dismally in their efforts though. They've also been hit with public outcry...

Did you know that back in 1974 all genetic engineering experiments were banned because of public concern as to where it was leading?

The genetic industry held a conference and declared to the world that they were just trying to find cures for deadly diseases like cancer and this was the only way. They were only allowed to resume work on the back of this massive promise which was a lie.

Now we have gone from banning their experiments on fetuses to all

---

[52] https://www.ncbi.nlm.nih.gov/books/NBK26818/

[53] www.ncbi.nlm.nih.gov/books/NBK26818/

volunteering to be their human guinea pigs and the world is their oyster.

I found this story after I wrote this piece but want to add it in now as it shows just how bad this **'wall'** was that GM was said to have hit.

"Jesse Gelsinger was 18 years old when he volunteered for a clinical trial at Penn State to test the effect GT would have on a rare metabolic disorder called OTC Deficiency. Within hours of being infused with 'corrective genes' encased in weakened adeno-virus, Jesse suffered multiple organ failure, and days later, his blood almost totally coagulated, swollen beyond recognition and brain dead, he was taken off life support. His death caused the then booming field of Gene Therapy to grind to a quiet screeching halt. The head of PR at Penn State said: "Not sure what to tell you. We killed an 18 year old kid." [54]

"In the last 5 years, we have seen a series of human trials being approved. 2020 gives us a series of really promising results for the first set of trials. <u>What is the goal of CRISPR-CAS9 technology?</u> CRISPR truly has a limitless potential and for that reason, every major industry is investing heavily in it. From biofuel companies to people who sell illegal highs. We could see CRISPR-CAS9 having an impact on our lives at every level." – From A Complete Guide to Understanding Crispr Gene Editing. [55]

So only in the last 5 years have human trials been allowed and 2020 gives them their results? Is covid their big human genetic engineering trial? Obviously yes. Who gave them this permission to break all the rules made back in 1974 to allow them to continue? Is this why they needed an 'emergency' to bend those rules? I think so and that is why covid was rolled out in the first place but if you think this is the first time they've used this technology you'd be wrong. The first vaccine they produced in a gene lab was the HepB hailed as the first cancer vaccine. The very one that caused the disease they called AIDS which Fauci and Mikovits were in on. The next one was the HPV which was their first attempt at 'curing' cancer except it didn't cure anything did it? They can't cure cancer because they know it is not a disease so they plumped for the unproveable prevention route and this was their second attempt at a cancer vaccine, with dire consequences again.

---

[54] https://open.substack.com/pub/celiafarber/p/the-machine-model-of-biology-denial?utm_campaign=post&utm_medium=web

[55] https://www.mybiosource.com/learn/guide-understanding-crispr-gene-editing/

Let's regroup again back to the cell debris. We are told the mRNA is a short strand of genetic material which tells the cell how to mix all the amino-acids to make a specific protein. If we have a blueprint why do we need these smaller bits of info and where do they supposedly come from? If they are just a strip of different chemicals how on earth do they do all the things they claim? From what they are claiming it's like saying a snip of a hair from my head can do double and triple salco's while cooking the dinner. They are 'discovering' loads more supposedly different RNA's too every day. Just add a letter or two before RNA like an M for instance. The inside of a cell is starting to look like downtown Manhattan by the sounds of it. OR are they simply looking at loads of cell debris from cells killed by their processes in the lab and playing a weird guessing game at who can come up with the best story explaining what it might do?

I found this gem of a paragraph in a science article. [56]

> For many new ncRNAs that are still being discovered, the function seems a bit more questionable. Many scientists are questioning whether assuming function because of existence is Panglossian. Some of these RNAs might just exist as a by-product of another process!

Guess what Panglossian means? Extreme optimism.

Yes it does look like science is fooling itself. Apart from everything they've seen of cells under the totally alien landscape of an electron microscope these cells are always grown in tissue cultures.

Harold Hillman pointed out that the cells in a tissue culture have "significantly different morphology, biochemistry, and environment than the cells from which they came." Meaning all in all they might as well be looking at a lump of dog turd to describe the workings of a human cell. NONE of it can be believed because the fantastical story they have concocted goes against everything we see in nature which is always simple and perfectly sensible.

Harold Hillman tried to stop this nonsensical storyline back in the 1970's providing evidence that our model of the cell was completely incorrect and used an old proverb as the intro to his book...[57]

---

[56] www.scienceabc.com/pure-sciences/what-does-rna-do-in-a-cell.html

[57] www.newbraveworld.org/modern-medicine-is-currently-in-dire-straights/

"It is easier to ride on the back of a tiger than to climb off it."

This Russian proverb, which appears at the beginning of Dr. Harold Hillman's last ever book, sums up the current state of our scientific establishment. Whether medicine, physics, or archaeology, all facets of scientific research rest on certain dogmas.

In essence, what this proverb is saying, is that it's easier to carry on perpetuating falsities than it is to admit you were wrong, drop everything and start again from scratch.

In my three weeks of delving into genetics I found no evidence of any of these things RNA is said to do. Since the PCR and assays were invented these are all that is used along with chemical reactions, a lot of math's and computer programs, all based on the original findings back in the early 1900's which looked at mutations and changes in fruit flies.

Along with all the high tech gear and AI they have moved from dead tissues to bacteria and fungi to do all the work for them. If they don't need the cells to do the gene splicing then surely it follows that it is the bacteria themselves that do it in the cells too? Bacteria are all killed when looking at cells under an electron microscope just like everything else, so they're claiming the bricks and mortar puts the fire out in a building and not the firemen, to use the old analogy again.

Apparently cells with no nucleus (so no DNA or chromosomes) like platelets in the blood, can produce proteins too – where do they get the recipe from? [58]

Activated platelets also release sticky proteins to help form the clot. A protein known as fibrin forms a mesh of threads that holds the plug together.

In the science labs working on genetics the only biological ingredients they use are bacteria and fungi (yeast). Remember fungi and yeast are just another form of the bacteria in the pleomorphic stages. They make genetics look very high tech with talk of snipping and editing but remember bacteria recycle cell debris, they also produce enzymes (which are a type of protein) which cause the different amino-acids which make up the proteins to break apart, just like they do in the digestive tract.

---

[58] www.medicalnewstoday.com/articles/314123#what-are-platelets

So from all this they deduce that RNA is as inanimate as DNA because it is just strings of acids, it doesn't DO anything, the BACTERIA are doing all the work in the lab AND in the cells. Another thing I saw mentioned a lot in the gene lab work was something called 'PLASMIDS'. They tell us that these are bacterial chromosomes. They use them as 'vectors' to 'deliver' drugs (RNA) into cells. The more I looked into these plasmids the more convinced I became that they were talking about bacteriophage again.

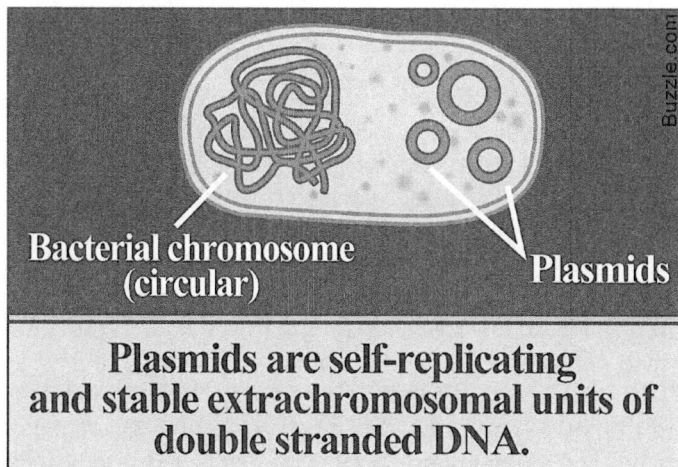

Bacterial chromosome (circular)

Plasmids

Plasmids are self-replicating and stable extrachromosomal units of double stranded DNA.

They based the whole of virology on these phages remember.

So plasmids are produced by bacteria and look like their description of a virus and they contain some genetic material. BINGO!

Plasmids are viruses are bacterio-phage and lets go one step further because in the pleomorphic graph what is the start and the end of the bacterial morphology? The somatid, also called a microzyma by Béchamp. It is immortal and contains all the information to start the whole process of life.

I've hinted at what I think this RNA could be already but then someone sent me a book in French about Béchamp's work and I translated this...

Bacteria are remarkable machine tools, intended to dismantle old/sick cells, cancers or scaffolds used to repair certain injuries. In this sense, it is fundamental to understand that we do not get germs from the outside. There is no biological warfare, says Béchamp. In an alkaline environment, microsomes assemble and manufacture bacteria. But if, on the contrary, the environment of the body returns to a neutral pH, the bacteria disassembles and the microsomes recover, moving freely.

Thus, depending on bio-electronic constants, temperature, presence or lack of oxygen and nutritional substances in the living environment, microsomes communicate with each other to form a certain germ, a mycelium, a micro bacteria that will be capable of fulfilling a certain mission.

A body does not get infected by contagion – bacillus or bacteria are built on the spot, when needed, to destroy damaged cells or tissues and to evacuate waste. Diseases of so-called 'pathogenic' germs are healing processes. They don't become serious unless important nutrients are missing.

For example, in the case of tetanus, microsomes build tetanic bacillus in deep muscle injuries caused by wounds or burns in an anaerobic environment (no oxygen). Their mission is to evacuate damaged cells and to rebuild new tissues. But this work requires a lot of energy and generates waste. In the absence of vitamin C, these wastes becomes toxic and trigger the famous spasms of tetanus.

It has been shown on several occasions that IV injection of magnesium chloride stops the spasms in half an hour. Alternatively, the injection of vitamin C brings healing in two or three minutes.

Microsomes are absolutely remarkable considering they can transform into other forms of living matter. They are complementary to each other, autonomous, specific, intelligent and responsible. They always do what's best for the body. But for this we need to provide them with the elements indispensable to their lives and their functioning – air, food, vitamin C (fresh fruit and veg).

Microlysis (e.g. E.coli) are capable of reproducing at very high speed and in very large numbers. They are not invaders or war aggressors. They feed and metabolize certain substances through a digestion mechanism. They need sugar, proteins, fatty materials and trace elements. They are living entities. They dismantle and remove waste. These entities made by microsomes can be dismantled, to atomic/chemical level again.

Microzymas are almost eternal (except for brutal destruction, through extreme processes – cremation, soaking in formaldehyde or pure acid). They can go into hibernation, partially dehydrated. Thus, live microsomes were discovered in fossils 12 million years old.

Microsides are specific to each individual and are likely responsible for the transmission of hereditary characters.

"Properties of microsome sickness, a rehearsal for life — Microsomes" – Antoine Béchamp. [59]

RIGHT so now we've sorted out that whole mess let's look afresh at the mRNA shots and the covid story…

The big topic on everyone's lips now is this SPIKE PROTEIN. We know they have no virus so there is no spike from any imaginary virus. This FACT that we know there is no spike protein IN the shots makes these shots a fraud. They are using the word 'vaccine' as a cover story and claiming the gene shot works like their vaccine theory because they can then be protected under the vaccine act from any litigation for the damage they are causing. Doubled with that they get to conduct their massive experiment on the back of an emergency pandemic rule permitting an experimental vaccine for a made up disease. This is double fraud. They really have pulled out all the stops this time. They are saying the 'SPIKE PROTEIN' is a poison/toxin.

I talk about Arthus and his dabbling with 'poison proteins' in the chapter 'Anaphylaxis'. So what are they? When Arthus was playing with them they were venom from snakes and later Richet played with jellyfish venom. They were playing with INJECTIONS of these 'poison proteins'.

The supposed deadliest of all 'poison proteins' is said to be Botulinum toxin. So how come people volunteer to have this stuff injected into their faces regularly? If it's so deadly why do they not drop dead? It does seem to paralyze muscles locally but doesn't spread and kill the whole body. Neither do they shed proteins so causing others to have instant facelifts. Ingested protein poisons only seem to affect the digestive system so it would seem the poison is localized and does not spread like a so-called virus is supposed to. Even though they claim extreme deadliness they can only affect the direct tissues they come in contact with. So far so good.

Could THIS be what their gain of function experiments have been trying to fix? I delved a bit deeper into 'poison proteins' but couldn't find much more of interest so ended up on general 'poisons' and while looking at the Britannica website I found this paragraph. [60]

---

[59] http://arhiva.formula-as.ro/2010/944/la-frontierele-stiintei-84/boala-o-repetitie-pentru-viata-microzimele-13108

[60] https://www.britannica.com/science/poison-biochemistry

Classification based on chemical activity

Electrophilic (electron-loving) chemicals attack the nucleophilic (nucleus-loving) sites of the cells' macromolecules, such as deoxyribonucleic acid (DNA), producing mutations, cancers, and malformations. Poisons also may be grouped according to their ability to mimic the structure of certain important molecules in the cell. They substitute for the cells' molecules in chemical reactions, disrupting important cellular functions. Methotrexate, for example, disrupts the synthesis of DNA and ribonucleic acid (RNA).

Some of this is obviously assumed and cause and effect being swapped around but basically they're saying that some poisons can cause mutations, yes we saw that with Thalidomide but what does it have to do with DNA? Nothing as these 'mutations' do not get inherited. People damaged by Thalidomide can have perfectly formed babies. How do poisons 'mimic'? They obviously don't so let's say they cause a reaction which damages the cell. Much simpler. Electron loving would imply a change in pH would occur, this would affect proteins produced. I didn't know what Electrophilic meant so looked it up and looky here. [61]

Electrophile, in chemistry, an atom or a molecule that in chemical reaction seeks an atom or molecule containing an electron pair available for bonding. **Electrophilic** substances are Lewis acids (compounds that accept electron pairs), and many of them are Brønsted acids (compounds that donate protons).

Examples of electrophiles are hydronium ion (H_3O+ from Brønsted acids), boron trifluoride (BF_3), aluminum chloride ($AlCl_3$) and the halogen molecules fluorine (F_2), chlorine (Cl_2), bromine (Br_2) and iodine (I_2).

Lots of those 'poisons' are pretty common in our day to day lives I'd say so maybe we can conclude that poison is not only in the dose but also in the vicinity. Maybe like weeds are just plants/wild herbs growing in the wrong place, these chemicals only become poisonous when they are in the wrong place as well as how much of it gets there. We also know we can become tolerant to an extent to these poisons in small doses. But not to proteins? Why are they treated differently?

---

[61] https://www.britannica.com/science/electrophile

Remember the anaphylaxis process? We still never worked out why that happens or how. I also found out that proteins can change their shape and function according to the environment and it seems to have a lot to do with pH and electrical charge. The pH measurement is actually ALL about the positive or negative charge of things. So the optimal pH is slightly alkaline which is a slight positive charge. Even though the sciences know this the biology side largely ignores it and treats the body like a chemical soup. It makes me wonder if all that 'junk DNA' they can't understand is nothing to do with recipes for proteins and chemicals and where the real stuff is. I'm reminded of a scene from the film The Fly where the scientist has to try and program the essence of life into his computer and his girlfriend tries to explain it to him but can't either.

Back to the lab...

So this 'spike protein' that they want our cells to manufacture, was it to be a poison protein? Well we know for damn sure it didn't come from a virus so where did they get the idea for it? From poison proteins and Arthus and anaphylaxis? Did they MAKE it? CAN they make it?

From what Malone told us, yes they have a synthetic protein 'on the shelf' so we can only guess what it is hoped to do from their objectives. Sterilization seems to be their main aim and it just came out from autopsies that this protein is being found concentrated in dead subject's ovaries, at least that is what they claim. Are they making a protein which is a specific poison to specific cells? That would make sense so it would end up where it's supposed to be right? How do they know it is concentrated in those parts of the body? What test are they using to show this? PCR or Assays? Both bogus tests. Are they finding a specific protein in these places or is it, as always the damage caused there by the poison protein?

They have been swapping the words 'virus' and protein for some years now and their evidence of a virus is always the damage caused by their chemicals so it would follow that the same evidence is being claimed here too. What is this thing 'off the shelf'? From what I gather it's a string of letters and numbers from the 'gene bank' which is more or less just hundreds of recipes for making synthetic proteins.

Only our own proteins made by our own cells are welcome in the body it would seem. So even a human protein from someone else would be 'foreign'. How does the body deal with 'foreign proteins'? This is where their 'immune system' theory comes into play and they treat foreign proteins with the same story as germs and viruses. The 'immune system' story.

Just like they concocted viruses from thinking they were seeing things exploding out of bacteria (phage) I'm beginning to wonder if they are swapping these proteins for what they thought were viruses exploding out of cells which were actually just dead cells being dismantled. They based viruses on bacteriophages as I explained in 'Going Viral – A Recipe For Disaster' so are they just expanding on that storyline now with proteins? Are proteins to be the new viruses?

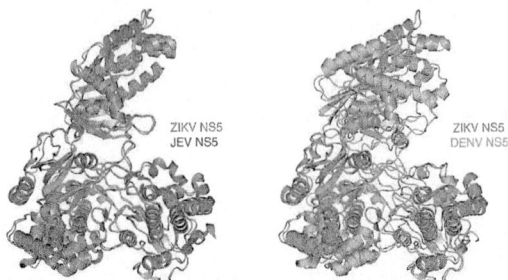

Structure of a Key Protein from the Zika Virus (Pfffff!) [62]

'Messenger' RNA is a figment of their imagination too but let's say that it is a 'drug' as they themselves describe it and a mixture of chemicals which is what all drugs are. This drug obviously can't provide our cells with any recipe to make a protein because it is 'foreign'. It can't get in. Just like in vaccine theory they need an adjuvant (a poison) to cause any reaction or rather to blast it in. They need a poison to deliver this poison into the cells. Our cells would never make a synthetic, foreign protein either as that would go against all the rules of nature.

They know this 'drug' can't gain access to our cells, they speak about it openly, this is why they say they used plasmids (or did in the past) to deliver the 'load'. That didn't work either because their virus theory is wrong and plasmids are not viruses anyway. They have used the old immunity card too to pretend they need to 'cloak' the drug so our bodies defense system won't see it.

The whole story of these shots is geared to pretending they are vaccinating us against a killer virus and the truth couldn't be further

---

[62] https://als.lbl.gov/structure-key-protein-zika-virus/

from that.

The antibody tests are another smoke screen long used in the vaccine fantasy. They claim antibodies prove the vaccine works but antibodies also DO NOT EXIST.

They are globulins and they are non-specific. That means the old theory that we make specific antibodies to specific germs is nonsense and they know this for sure because they know there are only a few different ones according to them. They are just proteins which clump together around toxins which can't be processed by enzymes (also proteins).

Compare it to throwing a blanket over a fire to put it out. So the appearance of globulins signifies ANY kind of poisoning which the body is having trouble processing. NOT a specific marker for any specific virus or germ nor any indication of 'immunity' which was clearly exposed by the HIV fiasco.

It seems they've been struggling to put that little nugget back into the box since they let it out.

Proof Fauci is a clown.

I watched a couple of painful videos about a scientist called Robert Malone who claims to be the inventor of this mRNA technology. Apart from the obvious chip on his shoulder over probably not getting a Nobel prize, his whining does reveal quite a lot about this whole gene/vaccine swap game they've pulled.

First I was struck by how little he seemed to understand about biology as he claimed they thought the ingredients from the shot would 'stay in the arm'. WHAT?!!

He reminded me of Judy Mikovits and her whining about being ousted from the old HIV game and how she exposes more than she thinks. I made copious notes from his interview with Smell Bigtree but will try to compact so much bullshit into hopefully a few nuggets.

Malone explains that he was working on vaccines at the Salk institute when a friend in genetics told him they 'hit a wall'.

I remember talking about this wall before and he explains what the wall was. They couldn't get the cells to 'express' the foreign proteins at all. That was the great wall genetic science hit. They thought it was our immune system and they couldn't work out how to get round it. They'd tried to 'fix' children with 'no immune system'.

Do you remember the 'Boy in a Bubble?

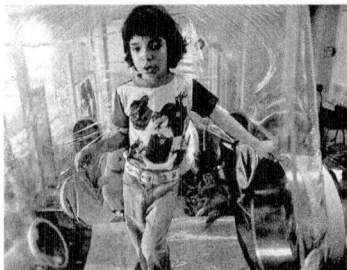

It's blatantly obvious to some of us that he was vaccine damaged and became a human lab rat for the genetics industry. All they did in the end was give the poor kid leukemia.

They also failed miserably with a cure for cystic fibrosis and never could find a way to cure cancer as they'd promised but they sure could induce it. [63]

So as I've explained, vaccines were struggling (particularly at the Salk institute as they had killed loads of kids with their polio vaccine and were now persona non grata) and genetics had hit a wall so these two muppets thought why not get together and we can sneak the non-working gene therapy in through the back door of the vaccine industry. It was a purely financial and political maneuver. Nothing to do with saving mankind.

He let slip that 'protein causes the immunity' so either he is thick or he's gone off script and revealed that they know there are no viruses and that proteins can induce an immune response (remember anaphylaxis). He also went on to state that the shots cause ADE.

I already told you that is science-waffle for anaphylaxis. So he exposed that they know this too.

He said that the 'spike protein' (he talked about 'Spike' a lot, like it was a friend of his) is a **"biologically active protein, it has effects, it modulates the immune system."** Now firstly that last bit is bull but how can he say this with such conviction unless he holds a patent on it? Or is it a euphemism for one of the 'drugs' they've developed called 'Spike'. He also stated his friend 'Spike' can open the blood-brain barrier. The best quote for me though was this: **"NIH engineered the spike off the shelf."** Off the shelf implies they got it from the gene bank, where all the patents are, for ingredients to make synthetic proteins (not viruses) and it would have been on the gene bank already BEFORE covid was launched.

---

[63] www.genecards.org/cgi-bin/carddisp.pl?gene=BCL5

HERE IS YOUR MADE IN A LAB VIRUS, oops protein.

He said these are 'first generation mRNA shots' and that no toxicology studies have been done, yet he then slipped in **"mice lie, monkeys mislead, only human data is relevant."** Which us antivivisectionists already knew but he is openly stating that covid IS THE TOXICOLOGY STUDY! Wow.

Malone is 'in the business of repurposing drugs' out of his own mouth, and works for the FDA which he said is 'not independent of political pressure' and Department of Defense. Well he certainly has repurposed vaccines and gene therapy hasn't he?

I wonder though how Gates managed to wheedle into this cushy little arrangement, there's no mention of him at all…no hang on, he did mention Moderna. During the original inventing he says there were patent battles for this new 'idea' of his between Moderna and BioNTech for recipes produced by him at Salk and the others working in the cancer field.

There we are, Gates was sticking his fingers in the pie right up to his elbows, yes. Most of the rest of his babble was just 'junk DNA' and of course pushing the bogus 'cure' for covid being some parasitic poison. So many people are buying that crap too even if they don't believe in covid they think it will placate the believers. All it does though is send everyone running back to the people who cause all this sickness in the first place with their poisons.

It drives me insane, the pure insanity of it all.

A Romanian friend on Facebook wrote this and it basically says it all in a nutshell.

"I don't believe in the bio-nano-tech manipulation thing that so called scientists brag about. What I think, is that these 'vaccines' contain certain 'toxins' that have already been tested on prisoners, orphans, mental[ly] sick and homeless people. My opinion is that the top producers and doctors in the so called research, claim anti-covid vaccines are experimental…just to provide a public excuse for the dramatic side effects occurring in case[s] of some of the vaccinated. However, the idea that the world 'scientists' have the scientific and technological ability to manipulate at bio-nano level, in my opinion is [a] disinformation so that they can appear in the eyes of the popular masses as semi-gods of intelligence and knowledge.

I believe that especially in the bio-medical field… all the so-

called advances in knowledge of the effects of toxins in vaccines and pharma-chemical medicines, are only done through uninterrupted clinical tests on defenseless people. So...how could they reveal this to the public...without compromising themselves? So the so called bio-medical researchers misinform and manipulate to give people the impression that they hold astonishingly advanced scientific and technological capabilities ...although in reality, with their poisons they cannot heal even a trivial cold." – N. Nedelcu.

Compare all this with what Moderna THINKS it can do with our bodies (bearing in mind this is Gates' computer company). 'Moderna claims they can program people like computers.' [64]

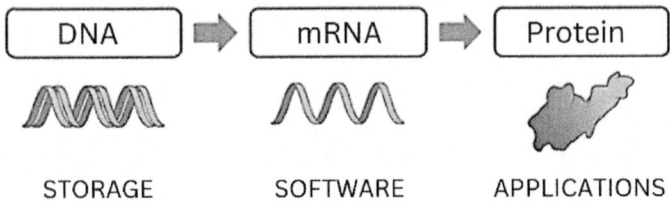

| DNA | mRNA | Protein |
| STORAGE | SOFTWARE | APPLICATIONS |

Is it correct to say that who controls the Protein Biosynthesis (the production/programming of proteins) controls life?

So to conclude and wrap this up...

Back to Harold Hillman who said **"two thirds of scientific work in biology since 1945 is fraud, led by secretiveness, dishonesty, hunger for money/fame, lack of proper equipment and compartmentalization in science."**

I think we have pretty much covered all that here, yes.

Now if they can't make any of this stuff work do you really think they can make trans-humans using this technology? I would take a stab at NO which is why I'm not delving into the nanotech at all.

It's all drawing board stuff but this experiment only concludes they can't make it work in practice so it's a mass cull dressed as a vaccine for a manufactured fake disease. If they can sterilize some of us that would be an added bonus but I doubt it is caused by their genetic experiments, it's just a side effect of the poisoning.

---

[64] thanks to: https://hive.blog/corona/@captainklaus/moderna-and-life-as-an-app-they-can-program

Sci-Fi or Sci-Fact?

Since I wrote my article on the AMINO AGE more scare mongering has come to light and I've been asked many questions by people who are still worried they can somehow 'catch' something from the unfortunates who have been already jabbed.

I know it was a complicated mission to try and explain what really goes on in these gene manipulation labs and maybe I did not simplify things enough. I do try. For those who did not get it I will try and outline the basic fraud I'm attempting to uncover and try to lift the veil finally on this nonsense. One of the things that keeps coming up is the 'magneto' effect, why it is happening and how does it affect us.

I looked into some of the scientific papers on the techniques they are using but more importantly WHY they are using these magnetic particles. The why is more important because it reveals the underlying mistake they are trying to overcome.

You see when I look at a paper, apart from having to learn new terminology to understand new research (along with new gobbledygook), certain sentences jump out and shout at me because of what we have already learned and debunked.

Here's an example from a paper on 'superparamagnetic nanoparticle delivery of DNA vaccine'. [65]

"The efficiency of delivery of DNA vaccines is often relatively low compared to protein vaccines. The use of superparamagnetic iron oxide nanoparticles (SPIONs) to deliver genes via magnetofection show promise in improving the efficiency of gene delivery both in vitro and in vivo."

Think about that first line. (Notice no mention of viruses at all). What problem are they trying to overcome? OK I'll tell you. They are basing all this 'gene insertion' research on the notion that **'viruses'** inject DNA into the cells forcing the cells to reproduce that DNA, remember? We know this is complete nonsense.

They concocted that story from seeing still electron microscope pictures of dead/poisoned/dying cells looking like a bomb site (that they caused) and concluded they had exploded and that the debris was new copies of DNA from an imaginary virus. Pure fantasy. They admit

[65] https://pubmed.ncbi.nlm.nih.gov/24715289/

their DNA (not virus) vaccines do not work but can't fathom why.

The old quote we often see is "scientists are baffled". Yeh, they are always baffled because they are lost in their own forest of wrong assumptions.

Secondly they admit that 'proteins' seem to work much better. Yes we have spoken about this foreign protein problem twice now and the old anaphylaxis reaction which they take to be the 'immune system' working. Ask yourself this though, why would the body react to a foreign protein but not as much to foreign DNA? I'll tell you again, because DNA (if it exists) is inert (in that it doesn't do anything so is harmless) whereas proteins are biological and do have functions and in the wrong place are not welcome and can be toxic. The body must deal with them which produces symptoms we can see and feel which they assume again is the 'immune system' working.

So this paper and many others I've been sent (along with scare-mongering video's by people who've watched too many sci-fi movies) are talking about and hinting at the old problem of getting our cells to take up DNA or RNA and replicate it. They can't do it in other words. This is why they have pumped so much money into 'gain of function' research. They are trying desperately to make their virus theory a fact but can't because it is wrong.

All the cell lines they use in their research are dividing cells like cancer cells or embryonic cells because, remember I told you, these are the only cells they've seen dividing and replicating the chromosomes. The magical never-seen DNA is said to be inside the chromosomes. Chromosomes are what genetics is all about and what classical genetics looked at, in other words hereditary genetics. 'DNA'/chromosomes are only replicated during reproduction and in real 'active' cancer cells. If it happened already in normal cells then why would they be trying so hard to **make** it happen? Maybe because it doesn't and won't, no matter how hard they try because the theory is just plain wrong.

So in short, our cells cannot be forced to replicate a synthetic, computer born protein. I believe this SPIKE PROTEIN story was a complete red herring to divert attention from the real ingredients.

Cancerous cells are a whole other subject which I've covered in the chapter 'What If Cancer Is Not A Disease But A Cure?' and in a talk I did with Sallie O'Elkordy years ago.

The whole gene therapy field has worked with cancer cells extensively and they haven't managed to harness that process either because they do not understand it even after years of searching. One thing they HAVE cottoned onto though is the 'energy' factor.

This is why they have turned to these nano-magneto particles BUT again they don't understand the energy/biology connection yet. Many alternative practitioners do understand it though like Chinese medicine (Ying Yang, chi and acupuncture are all bio-energetic protocols). The problem with that is there is no money in it, nothing they can patent and sell so they have to use chemistry (alchemy). Their materialistic brains cannot fathom that healing is free for all and inbuilt in our own biology. They can never harness that while profiting from and controlling us so they are stuck in their own forest of wrong-think, scrabbling about in the dirt looking for more ways to make us sick and profitable.

There has also been a lot of talk about GRAPHENE lately so I went and had a look at what that is and if it can do what it says on the truthers tin again. What is 'graphene'? Again they like to baffle us with scientism but really it is just a form of carbon.

Difference between Graphite and Graphene:

The key <u>difference</u> between <u>graphite</u> and <u>graphene</u> is that <u>graphite</u> is an allotrope of carbon having a higher number of carbon sheets whereas <u>graphene</u> is a single carbon sheet of <u>graphite</u>. <u>Graphite</u> is a well-known allotrope or carbon. [66]

Graphite is what they put in pencils. I saw a cool little video of a man showing how you can make graphene from a pencil. He scribbled a dot on a piece of paper with a pencil, then stuck a piece of sellotape over the dot, pulled it off and said that was a thin layer of graphite, then he again stuck another piece of sellotape to the first piece and pulled them apart again and explained now he had a nano layer of graphite which he said is now 'graphene'. So it's just the thinnest layer possible of carbon. Ta-da!. How scary was that? No, not scary at all is it? It brings a whole new meaning to the old magic pencil story.

Does it belong inside the body though? I would say a big fat NO. Is it a protein? Also a NO but none of these shots' ingredients belong in the body. How does the body deal with an injection of nano-graphite (carbon)? I don't know and I'm not sure they do either but I'm pretty sure it poses no threat to anyone who isn't getting it injected into them

---

[66] www.differencebetween.com/difference-between-graphite-and-graphene/

so I'd say the jabbed are again no threat from so called 'shedding'.

All the talk of vaccines being developed that can vaccinate the unvaccinated is pure fantasy too. If they've never managed to make even one vaccine work it's a big step to claim they can make a massive jump from ineffective to infective let alone effective.

They do seem to be trying to mess with our bio-field with all these magneto nano-products which means we are going to have to learn more about this always considered 'fringe' and 'woo' medicine and openly mocked because behind those closed doors THEY are taking it very seriously actually.

If you want to find out about how our bodies are 'energy' and 'frequency' based look at the work of Eileen Day McKusick and be blown away. Lanka says our bio-information (the DNA blueprint in other words) is NOT in the nucleus of our cells at all but in our bio-field, the 'aura' the 'consciousness'. Rupert Sheldrake long ago hypothesized our memories were not stored in our brains but outside of our bodies in the 'consciousness'.

The fields of 'Energy-Medicine' are being heavily mocked and diverted from because they are such a threat to many of their new 'weapons', 5G being one which may be used for targeting our bio-energy. German New Medicine or 'New Biology' is a threat to the cancer business and also looks at illness from an energy/frequency perspective. Also homeopathy was always about an energy field/memory held in water or pill form.

A lot of people think science is exactly what they see in sci-fi films and teLIEvision PROGRAMMING. We've had all the CONTAGION films bombarding us with the nonsense of antibodies and searching for that one immune person, now we have gene-manipulation programming like one I watched called Biohackers. Programs like this literally program us to believe they can do all this fantastical stuff with their gene technology but it's a lot of wishful thinking and fantasy. It is far from truth and the reality of what's going on in these labs. It's also a form of marketing to keep the money rolling in while never actually delivering their promises of cancer cures and everlasting life, just fantasy scenarios.

Gene 'therapy' will never deliver any cures for anything because just like germs were not killing us and viruses were the invisible new fantasy enemy, genes are also NOT the cause of any diseases therefore they cannot be a cure. Their man-made strings of amino-acids which they patent and want to inject into you are their own fantasy chemical concoctions of what they think genes are or at least what they want us to believe in and buy.

Speaking of patents, an interesting interview was aired of Dr. David Martin giving his testimony to Reiner Fuellmich and his crew which was very interesting in that it exposes what they have patented and when. One in particular was the famous 'SPIKE PROTEIN'.

In his testimony he states that this particular protein they call 'Spike' is a computer simulated sequence of amino acids and it was patented in 2008!!! So not 'novel' at all and certainly not real. Remember nothing in nature can be patented. If you think you know enough now about patents and computer modelling then watch this man wipe the floor with these so-called life-saving, cure-finding sciences. They actually are criminals and you've been had. [67]

"…we took the reported gene sequence, which was reportedly isolated as a novel coronavirus – indicated as such by the ICTV (the International Committee on Taxonomy of Viruses of the World Health Organization). We took the actual genetic sequences that were reportedly 'novel' and reviewed those against the patent records that were available as of the spring of 2020. And what we found, as you'll see in this report, are <u>over 120 patented pieces of evidence to suggest that the declaration of a novel coronavirus was actually entirely a fallacy</u>."

(There's a partial transcript of the above interview on Truthcomestolight.com).

Addendum

After I published this on my blog it seems someone else was coming to similar conclusions and I was asked to include a link to an online call with Argentine geneticist Dr. Luis Marcelo Martinez being interviewed by Pedro Moreno in the program Integrantes. If nothing else it's a prime example of 'scientists are baffled' again.

At least this guy is asking the right questions though. [68]

And I found an interesting article on the science of genetics which exposes a whole lot of the lies we've been fed in the public arena about

---

[67] https://odysee.com/@dharmabear:2/David-Martin-deposition-Reiner-Fuellmich-July-9-2021:2?r=BgSpgR6UE73qW3b8FEgK6N2oj9vhfjB3

[68] https://www.orwell.city/2021/07/the-spike-protein-is-graphene-oxide.html

this 'science'. Recommended reading. [69]

I've also came across another excellent blog on DNA which goes into the processes used to 'prove' the existence of it (or not). Great to see more people picking their pseudo-science apart now. [70]

PROTEINS, BACTERIA AND TECHNOCRACY

"Where do you get your protein from?"

This is a question every vegan gets asked regularly and is also answered just as regularly but being me I always like to go a bit deeper.

In my research on germ theory I learned that germs, rather than being an enemy which attacks us, are actually essential to the workings of our bodies. Most 'terrain theory' proponents claim we have 'good and bad bacteria' and that balance is key. This theory still has one foot in the camp of 'bacteria cause disease'. I would take it one step further and say we have healthy or unhealthy bacteria meaning the health of the bacteria is what is important.

Healthy bacteria = good. Unhealthy bacteria = bad.

This theory is also mirrored in modern plant science, particularly the organic sector. They preach about 'feeding the soil and not the plants'. So what are they talking about? How does soil need 'food'?

Dead soil (desertification) which nothing grows in is devoid of life, it is devoid of BACTERIA! They are saying feed the bacteria in the soil/dirt. Soil without bacteria is just dirt. Plants do not grow in dirt hence plants need bacteria to grow.

As all our 'knowledge' (be it right or wrong) of human biology has stemmed from plant science (genetics were discovered by a botanist, the first virus was claimed to be discovered in tobacco plants) then it follows the 'as above so below' discoveries in plants also cross over to human biology. We also need bacteria to grow and to be healthy.

When I looked into this new mRNA technology and it's use of CRISPR technology I was surprised to learn they use bacteria to manipulate the genetic codes (as covered in chapters 'The Amino Age' and 'Protein, Spikes and Bio-Weapons'). They also use yeast extensively for many things and if we add in the terrain theory again of yeast being

[69] https://www.medicdebate.org/node/2208

[70] https://criticalcheck.wordpress.com/2021/12/15/dna-discovery-extraction-and-structure-a-critical-review/

just another form in the pleomorphism of bacteria then it is still. [71]

So where am I going with this? Well in 'The Amino Age' I hinted that there is more to bacteria than they have been telling us. They might not just be the garbage men of the body, their role(s) might be much bigger and more important than that.

We have been told that it is our cells that produce proteins by reading parts of the DNA in the cell signaled by messengers (mRNA). But those things are not living, they are crystalline so cannot 'do' anything on their own. They cover this by telling us ribosomes in the cell do the work which they say are RNA mixed with proteins which sound like their description of 'viruses' but they 'live' in the cells.

If they are living and do that work then they are more than just RNA and proteins. I would call them microbes or BACTERIA.

RIBOSOME

Ribosomes, also called Palade granules, are macromolecular machines, found within all cells, that perform biological protein synthesis. Ribosomes link amino acids together in the order specified by the codons of messenger RNA molecules to form polypeptide chains.

Another thing they say lives in the cell are mitochondria which they say provides the 'food' for the cell by chemistry.

MITOCHONDRION

A mitochondrion is a double-membrane-bound organelle found in most eukaryotic organisms. Mitochondria use aerobic respiration to generate most of the cell's supply of adenosine triphosphate, which is subsequently used throughout the cell as a source of chemical energy.

Which reminded me of this paper I found a while ago. I found the title hilarious, makes you wonder who are the amateurs really.

Bacteria Find Work As Amateur Chemists

"New evidence demonstrating that certain bacterial strains can synthesize semiconductor nanocrystals through endogenous pathways may open the door to new strategies for the biosynthesis of unnatural materials and compounds." [72]

I was beginning to see a pattern here pointing to bacteria doing ALL the work in the body and not just garbage collection. Something they

---

[71] www.life-enthusiast.com/articles/pleomorphism-gaston-naessens/
[72] www.nature.com/articles/nmeth0105-6a

have been hiding from us for a long time so as not to upset the apple cart which feeds the whole medical sciences – that bacteria are the enemy.

I wasn't absolutely sure of what I was hypothesizing until I watched a film about the dairy industry in New Zealand called MILKED. I wouldn't normally have watched this but because it was New Zealand (where my sister lives) and the description peeked my interest. It didn't tell me much I didn't already know but then at 1:13 mins in I hit the jackpot! [73]

A company called RETHINKX has developed a method of producing milk 'without the cow' using 'precision fermentation processes'. What was germ theory and terrain theory born from? Fermentation experiments by Béchamp and his nemesis Pasteur. What does the job of fermentation? BACTERIA.

Now we are seeing the proof that BACTERIA MAKE PROTEINS themselves. NOT our cells. Without BACTERIA our bodies on their own cannot synthesize proteins from amino-acids. The BACTERIA build them – hence the bacteria build us or at least they build the building blocks of us. The proteins.

Bacteria also breakdown proteins which means they are our digestive system not just a part of it. All that 'science' (from the 1800's too) about the stomach producing hydrochloric acid is utter nonsense and was debunked by Dr. Robert O'Young. So next time somebody asks where I get my protein from I can tell them – from my bacteria. Look after your bacteria because they are keeping you alive, not killing you at all. Also think about what 'antibiotics' are doing to your body next time you're told you need to poison all the bacteria in your body.

---

[73] https://join.waterbear.com/milked

AREN'T WE HUMAN AFTER ALL?

"A lot of what is presented as 'the science' in modern medicine is woefully lacking and probably always has been. This has resulted from starting off on the wrong track, and when we start off on the wrong track, every move we make from then on takes us farther and farther off track.

In medical science, it has led to pure theory becoming the dogma of today's medicine. Why did this happen? It was inevitable. It resulted from medical science consciously leaving out of the study of human disease a few rather important things: the human psyche (thoughts and emotions), the human energy system, the human connection to the whole of the universe.

Instead, it chose to narrow its so-called medical science down to a view of the human body as a machine. And from that faulty basis it proceeded to look at disease as the breaking down of the parts of the machine, the solutions to which are mostly drugs (which just happen to crank out huge bucks for the medical conglomerates controlling medicine today). True science makes sense. It is understandable to the common person. Furthermore, its conclusions are verifiable.

Yet, here we are. Instead of having a medical system that most people would be able to understand, because it actually makes sense and could be taught appropriately from the lower grades and up, we have a so-called science that is full of errors because so much of it is actually made up. To cover up for this, it contains a lot of long words and names to keep the public dependent on the "experts" for answers, thus turning off their instincts in the face of nonsense that is being preached or prescribed to them.

I believe that what we are seeing happen right now, all around the world, is the inevitable end of the line for such a faulty system. At the very least, it is a crossroads. It could mean the end of the human race as it has been known since the beginning of humankind. Or it could be a wake-up call and an opportunity to recognize that what we are witnessing – and have been witnessing for a long time, now – is the end of a civilization.

If this awakening can occur among great numbers of us all over the planet, we will be given the chance to stop what is happening now and, using our own inner guidance, create a world the likes of which has not been known since the ancient

Vedic civilization. I have faith that this is what is about to happen in our beautiful world.

But it will only happen if people awaken from the trance they've been put in, start questioning and thinking independently, and make a firm decision to create a world for themselves, and the following generations, that we can finally love." – From 'Why I Have Turned To The New Biology And Medicine' by Joan Hughes.

My friend wrote that and it kind of ties all my previous articles together nicely. She gets it, but this time I'm delving into transhumanism. After learning about genes and a bit about DNA it's the next logical step to understanding what is going on and why.

I ended up watching lots of videos on the subject and gleaned what I could and started joining some dots again. I don't believe they are trying to make us into cyborgs as some people think. That doesn't make much sense. Actual robots would be much more compliant and cheaper. They could be experimenting on us to make themselves into cyborgs though as they do seem obsessed with 'eternal life' and it would be the ultimate materialistic experience.

We do know they want to 'upload' our minds into this cloud thing. The quantum computer to run this cloud is called 'D-Wave'. They like to put everything in plain sight for us which is why instead of going through the Greek alphabet from A-Z which would be logical, they have instead called the 'effects of the shots' the Delta Wave. Delta wave is also a frequency our brains emit when we are in deep sleep. Get it? Following on from D-wave the next one waiting in the wings is called the MU wave.

First I thought of the Mumu Land song from the 80's which came from a trilogy of books called The Illuminati Trilogy so thought I had it but then I heard of the tiniest chip they've managed to make. Barely the size of a piece of dust and it is called a MU-chip. Bingo. Maybe they HAVE put a chip in the jabs? Or maybe that's in the booster shot hence MU wave not being rolled out yet.

Just as they have done with genetic research although they can only relate to materialism so they correlate our minds with our material being, but are our minds entirely us? No.

Rupert Sheldrake has already demonstrated that our memories are not even stored in our brains, they are stored outside the body in the 'bio-field'. Our soul/bio-field extends out from our physical body, some see it as an 'aura' and it's said to extend to about 6 feet. This is not an exact science and with metrics I remember a lot of arguing over how far apart we should all be for their 'social distancing'. So what they want to upload are our material 'reactions' using Google algorithms. This is to be a 'global super brain', maybe our supreme leader in the New World Order.

They do like to emulate the Good Book, relive things from it or even bring things like Revelations into reality. This uploading to the cloud is an enactment of the Rapture but in materialistic form or is the rapture an analogy for this transhumanism? Are we being manipulated into enacting scenes from their bible? You may not believe in the bible but you can bet your socks they do most avidly.

The mind is not our soul/consciousness, it is only the materialistic dimension of ourselves. In fact it is the 'heart chakra' (whatever that might be) which new agers say is the key to our soul (or is it our DNA?). Is it a coincidence that the jabs are affecting men's hearts? Why men's hearts but women's nerves and ovaries? We need to look at the real data to see if I'm right, it's just what I've perceived myself. Women seem to be getting the wobbles where men seem to be having heart issues. Correct me if I'm wrong. Is this on purpose or accidental?

I'm reminded of the murals in Denver airport in which there are no men, only women and children in the apocalyptic scene.

So modern medicine treats us all like machines, modern genetics treats us like a chemistry lab and now transhumanists think our brain is our entirety. They always seem to fall short of the mark don't they? Some of these quantum scientists claim we are living in a computer simulation already but I think that is wishful thinking on their part and what they would like it to be.

The genetics industry has always run on a 'fake it till you make it' marketing policy and it would follow that the same applies to the transhumanists. They are telling us what they are wishing for.

THE STORY OF ADAM AND EVE [74]

Adam and Eve. The story has always intrigued me and I could never make sense of it until recently. I was lent a book written by a Catholic priest which I cannot remember the name of but it jolted me to think again. It pointed out that they couldn't have been the first humans made by God as it clearly says later in the bible that Cane left the

---

[74] www.getty.edu/art/collection/object/107TXP

Garden of Eden and went to find himself a wife.

So Adam and Eve were not alone, or the first, so who were they? The book also stated that the Catholic priest believed they were the first 'Israelites'. That it is the story of the Israelites only, which makes more sense now. The Old Testament is full of stories which do not fit with Christian values at all. What does fit though is Satanism. Animal and human sacrifice, more than one 'God', magic and spells.

So if we look at the story again with fresh eyes (which I recently did) more of the story makes sense.

I dabbled at first with the alien cloning theory, the rib being used to take the DNA but it was only Eve that was 'cloned'.

The 'Tree of Life' would be the Kabbalah which coincidentally (not) is still referred to AS The Tree of Life. OBVIOUSLY!

The snake is the devil or rather, was it his trouser snake and that apple is now his seed? He impregnated Eve to make himself in the flesh, mirroring the story of Jesus' conception. Cane was the devil's child. The Israelites are Lucifers chosen people. The bloodline of the illuminati is the bloodline from Cane.

Other stories about 'fallen angels' or the Nephilim breeding with humans fits in with this too. The elite are obsessed with inbreeding, trying to keep their bloodline pure but they cannot survive and procreate indefinitely without problems. They must hate having to turn to us for our genes to keep them going and by doing so muddying their pure bloodline.

All through history we, the ones outside the Garden of Eden, have been controlled by these 'spawn of Satan, good versus evil, dark versus light'. All the stories now fit. The Roman gods, the Egyptian mythology, Ayurvedic tales all begin to make sense of the fight for domination over us. The early Israelites worshipped Ba'al, remember the golden calf? The elites still do worship Ba'al. It's no secret any more.

I remember getting suckered in by the Zeitgeist films about 10 years ago in which they tried to say the story of the birth of Jesus was simply older stories rehashed. The birth of Horus as an example, but now I believe those stories were actually the Adam and Eve story rehashed.

The article 'Scientific Evidence That Adam and Eve Never Even Met Never Mated So What's The Story?' can be found on newsintact.com. [75]

But why am I talking of Adam and Eve and what does it have to do with our current situation or even transhumanism?

Well a lot actually. It was only when I delved into the transhumanist agenda that everything started to make sense. We always have to look at the history to see how we got here and Adam and Eve have always been postulated as 'clones'. Clones of what though? Those who do not believe in God prefer to think of it as an alien genetic experiment. That's fine, to me aliens are just demons and I think it's just biblical stuff dressed up in pseudoscience .

It also stated in Genesis somewhere that humans should only live for 120 years yet the descendants of Adam and Eve were listed as living for hundreds of years, so these were not products of God? Why did they stop living so long and what happened to the 'giant' children? Did the human DNA cancel out their demon/alien DNA down the generations? Is this what they are looking for, their original DNA?

Another thing that I couldn't get my head around was the 'we are energy beings' thing. We are just experiencing a 'material world'. This is our soul, the energy (some say we are light others say electric but it's all energy in material forms). Frequencies seem to be the key. Some frequencies seem to be bad and some good. Low and high frequencies. Low is bad, high is good. Is this our heaven and hell analogy? Back to the bible and Genesis "In the beginning was THE WORD."

So not light but sound. Everything sprang from a sound (hmm the 'Big Bang' ring any bells? I made a pun). The Illuminati are the illuminated ones, illuminated by the light of the Light Bearer (Lucifer), or given 'life' by their God. Biblical hints are written all over the place on this covid story, we can't ignore it.

Now let's link all this historical storytelling to what we've been trying to work out about DNA and why it is so important to our power-crazed 'elite', 'rulers', whatever you want to call the control freaks pulling the strings.

Is this DNA the receiver, translator from energy to matter? It has been referred to as Jacob's ladder which would be the thing that connects us to God/Source. It is not biological, it is more crystalline and is likened to a computer code in materialistic thinking. All these

---

[75] https://newsinstact.com/scientific-evidence-that-adam-and-eve-never-even-met-never-mated-so-whats-the-story-14013/

things fit with it being the connection between energy and matter. Our DNA is the program which makes our soul run our biological bodies. This is why it is so important and why everyone says this is a spiritual battle.

They've been collecting DNA since before the great covid drive, remember all the fuss about family trees and sending your DNA in to be analysed? Yup, they'd started collecting, then the PCR tests which look for specific bits of RNA.

Not sure what they were looking for there, maybe their own bloodline off shoots, bits of their own DNA, who knows?

Crispr/CAS9 is said to be a tool for 'hacking DNA' which is what they would love to do no doubt but I feel they are still faking it till they make it. I covered where they're at with that technology in the 'Amino Age' chapter. If they could hack our DNA they could theoretically cut us off from source, our souls. We would be like zombies which they also seem to be throwing at us constantly. If people have been chipped with the MU-chip it would certainly help with their planned social credit system. The chip works on a super low frequency which it emits (could this be the cause of the 'shedding' phenomena?) and which a simple gadget can pick up. It was said to be invented to tag shop items like clothing but that makes no sense does it? Sounds like a cover story. Just like their continued experimenting with genes used the cover story of finding cures when genes do not cause disease. Apparently these MU-chips are already in lots of so-called 'food' items.

As usual I'm leaving you with more questions than answers but this time I really don't know what they are trying to do exactly. We know they want eternal life, they had it once or near enough but they lost those 'genes' somewhere in the mix. I think they're trying to get it back and I think they're fighting a losing battle. Maybe they'll just have to plump for total control of everything on God's earth, making us all live in their hell with them. They obviously need us but not in these great numbers so a cull is obvious and underway.

I think historically we've been here before, as in done this before. The remnants are with us in stories like the Tower of Babel, Sodom and Gomora and Atlantis and Sumeria – advanced civilizations who went one step too far. Looks like they're about to overstep the mark once again and it will not end well.

Rinse and repeat…

EX-SPURTS – WHO DO YOU LISTEN TO?

The more they take the mickey out of 'conspiracy theorists' the more conspiracies are unleashed. I've been watching all the new ones cropping up and trying to glean what I can from the info deluge. What is factual and what is assumption. What are these 'crazy' 'conspiracy nuts' basing their findings on? Some of them are 'geneticists', immunologists, scientists and have had nothing to do with 'conspiracies' before except that they are part of one of the longest running conspiracies in modern history, whether they know it or not. Others are long time 'hard-nuts' in the game.

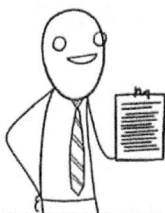

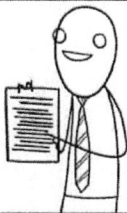

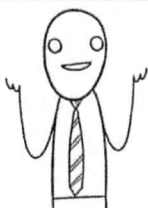

I've kind of socially distanced myself from ALL mainstream media for years now but in the last few years I've had to turn off even what I considered more relevant journalists and news sites because they seem (to me at least) to be just going round and round in circles too, picking at the small stuff, the crumbs of the MSM who are still playing the same broken-down record since March 2020. Masks, flu, skewed data, viruses, deaths, cases, tests and on and on ad nauseum.

I just can't fathom how people are still talking about the same stuff. I feel like I'm making headway then someone makes me listen again to Richie Allen and I find I'm having to run on the spot to wait for these people to catch up but they're not following. They've gone round the track again and some of us are already in another playing field altogether playing a new game.

For the last five years there was a big surge in those who thought the only way we can fight the science is to use the science. Peer review was the mantra and no layperson was allowed to have a view unless it had been 'peer reviewed' or they could back up what they say with some piece of paper. This 'scientism cultish-ness' was creeping into all sectors and movements. Effectively it became a form of gagging and censorship.

Basically it was saying if you are not qualified to understand the science your voice is irrelevant and I'm using the words 'qualified' and 'understand' in as sarcastic a tone as can be mustered here.

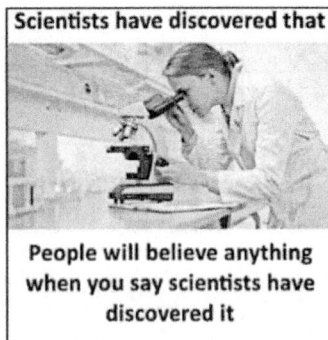

Scientists have discovered that

People will believe anything when you say scientists have discovered it

DOCTORS AND OTHER MEDICAL PROFESSIONALS

Are they really ex-spurts when it comes to a worldwide plandemic 'vaccine' marketing campaign?

Firstly MD's do less than 7 hours of spoon-fed reading on vaccines and most of that is studying the schedule, not ingredients nor anything relevant to safety or more importantly efficacy. When I say that most parents who do their own research into vaccines know more than any MD I am not joking. It is absolutely true. Once a doctor has finished his indoctrination/training from the literature he has been told to learn from, he will have no time to update or flesh out what he has learned from then on. Any updates come directly from pHarma reps and administration level. So if they are calling the covid shots 'vaccines' you can immediately switch off.

They haven't a clue in other words. You really are much better off listening to those pesky 'anti-vaxxers' everyone warns you about. Some of them are actual 'experts' and even qualified doctors and MD's.

SCIENTISTS

"All science is merely a means to an end. The means is knowledge. The end is control. Beyond this remains only one issue – who will be the beneficiary?" – from the book 'Silent Weapons for Quiet Wars'.

"I regard consensus science as an extremely pernicious development that ought to be stopped cold in its tracks. Historically, the claim of consensus has been the first refuge of scoundrels; it is a way to avoid debate by claiming that the matter is already settled. Whenever you hear the consensus of scientists agrees on something or other, reach for your wallet, because you're being had.

Let's be clear, the work of science has nothing whatever to do with consensus. Consensus is the business of politics. Science, on the contrary, requires only one investigator who happens to be right, which means that he or she has results that are verifiable by reference to the real world. In science consensus is irrelevant. What is relevant is reproducible results. The greatest scientists in history are great precisely because they broke with the consensus. There is no such thing as consensus science. If it's consensus, it isn't science. If it's science, it isn't consensus. Period." – Michael Crichton from a lecture at the California Institute of Technology, 2003

FRIENDS AND SOCIAL MEDIA

Well this about sums it all up. 😕 😑
"Why it's all but impossible for thinking humans to trust the government:
"Get the shot, and you won't have to wear the mask and you'll be protected … except you will need to wear one again and you won't be protected … still … until we say you don't have to anymore … but we might not, so wear it just in case … and you might need to add a booster so you REALLY won't have to wear the mask and you'll be protected … except you will need to when we say to, and you may not be protected … oh, and variant Z is here, so 2 weeks/6 ft/circuit breaker/new normal/stay inside/we are in this together."
If you let them get away with this nonsense, you can rinse, lather, and repeat it all for the rest of your life."

On this occasion ask yourself 'qui bono', who benefits? Are your friends making money by warning you about 'vaccines' and pHarma? Do they have a business selling their own 'snake-oil'? Or are they just trying desperately to save their loved ones from harm? A good friend wrote that she had 'read my stuff' and she 'didn't agree' BECAUSE she 'knew people' who had been sick.. I'm beginning to think some people are actually enjoying this. Why else would they turn a blind eye to the real remedy when it is shoved in their face? Is there such a thing as an addiction to allopathy? I know there is, I've seen people go willingly back time and again until their eventual death. Hypochondriacs who become self-proclaimed ex-spurts in the allopathic mantra and love to play the perpetual victim. They are the ones keeping the wheels on this gravy train turning. Like the last sentence of that post above, they will rinse and repeat with relish.

GOVERNMENT

Do I really need to explain this one? The word itself says it all. Latin explanation: Govern=to control, Ment=mind. Government is mind control and they are doing it so well. If you are listening to them you are truly hypnotized and the media is the hypnotic stage show. FEAR is their weapon of choice and the ammo is always a 'virus'. Their stage is the mainstream media. Without the virus they have no ammo to produce the fear which is why we have to prove there is no invisible bogeyman virus. It is the only real remedy.

Last week the CDC announced that PCR (which the whole plandemic has been based on) does not differentiate between flu and convid so they will be trashing it. Did this wake the stragglers up? It really should have shouldn't it? Those 'friends who got sick' all based on this bogus test. Maybe it's a case of not wanting to admit they've been duped. They've committed up to their necks and would rather sink in the quicksand than admit they've been conned. Yes I know there are people that will die for their cause which is noble if the cause is true. This cause though is virus theory which is based on lies, money, power, greed and genocide.

I have tried my best to expose the lies. I've been waiting for friends and family to leave the cult but they don't seem to want to. I know how they get people out of cults in real life, they kidnap them back. How do we do that on such a massive scale?

Answers on a postcard please...

VACCINES

INTERVIEW WITH AN 'ANTI-VAXXER'

Yes I know it's a dirty word and I cringe at using it too but not for the reason you might think. The term 'vaxxer' was made popular (and unpopular) by the 'Vaxxed' campaign and movie, started by Dr. Andrew Wakefield and his crew.

Now anyone would think this philosophy was brand new looking at it from outside of my world but actually the anti-vaccination movement has been around as long as vaccinations have been around and before that almost everyone was anti-inoculation which is what vaccines were born from.

The trouble with inoculation, apart from the damage it was causing, like deaths and disease (cough ... smallpox), was that it was unregulated. Anyone and his brother could go and scratch someone's poxes off and scratch them onto someone else. Just like butchers in the days of unregulated 'medisin' could perform the old cure-all of blood-letting. (That's basically stabbing you and letting you bleed for a bit). Yes, literally butchers, who sold dead animals.

So to halt the 'charlatans' making money and going around killing people, the powers that be saw a nice little earner so got their minion (a lowly freemason) Edward Jenner to come up with the genius plan of using cows pox pus instead of human pox pus, give it a fancy Latin name (Vacca means cow in Latin) vaccination, ban anyone else from doing it by patenting the process and banning inoculation. Ta-daaa, a great new business model for making pots of cash AND keeping the population down. You've gotta hand it to them. A genius plan which even I didn't spot until recently.

I spent 35 years trawling through 'science', listening to others talking about vaccines, immune systems, antibodies, ingredients, contagious diseases. It was a minefield of half-truths, half lies, tangents, mud-slinging and rabbit holes. It's any wonder I came out the other end with all my marbles intact. But I did.

After chewing on the 'science', which everyone seemed to think was the answer to everything, ignoring the fact that it had got us into this mess in the first place, I finally found the emperor of medical science actually was wearing no clothes. Not only was he naked but he'd forced us all to wear magical Latin specs so we couldn't actually see his naked ugly body jiggling down the main streets of every town and city in the 'civilized' world.

STILL the 'anti-vax' crew were biting everyone's ankles with the mantra of 'peer review', like it was some elixir of truth. 'Trust the science' they all cried until the whole world had to trust it too.

It is a very difficult task to break out of the cult of scientism just like any cult is. Many are still stuck in there with no hope of escaping.

The industry was on the run but the anti-vaxxers were still navel gazing. They should have picked up pace. No more picking at individual vaccines, exposing them individually which is time consuming and moves at snail-pace as the industry just makes new recipes, even mixing multiple recipes together as fast as we could pull them down. Remember how much fuss was made of a 3-in-1 like the MMR? That is so last year. Now they have 6-in-1's.

It was a losing game YET the anti-vaccine movement WAS gaining ground. We had them worried. They were so worried they even made new peer reviewed papers about 'vaccine hesitancy'. That was a goal to us, they were on the back foot.

THEN we got covid. Is this going to be an own goal for the vaccine industry? Never before have so many actually questioned what these cults are injecting into us. It could be an own goal yet the irony of the whole thing is that the covid shots ARE NOT EVEN VACCINES.

Just when we were starting to expose the whole basis of vaccines and even 95% of modern medicine by realising they had based it all on a false theory. Germs do not cause disease…

This has confused the anti-vaccine movement as having had their heads in the trough of germs, viruses, immune systems, and all that nonsense, we've suddenly been flung into the even more fairytale storyland of genetics.

This was another genius move on the oppositions part. They have not only moved the goalposts, they've changed their kit and moved the bloody playing field.

Multiple reasons for doing this, the main one being avoiding the long and arduous testing process and also litigation. They even get to ride on the massive reputation of 'vaccinating' built up over 200 years. They used a kind of Trojan Horse tactic to usher in a brand new technology and dressed up the naked emperor with a new fancy outfit including bells and whistles.

Now everyone is scrabbling about in the dark again until those of us who HAVE taken a look at this new outfit can somehow explain in plain English, what the flippin' heck is going on in those secret labs?

Now we have to listen to all the nonsense about bio-weapons, manmade viruses, gain of function and genomes until everyone is brought up to date on the new rules of their game.

I have written down everything I've so far come to understand. I don't think there is anything more to explain. It's all there already. Until the game gets rigged again…

This article was inspired by a devastating post I saw and which has personal implications. The one thing that may come out of this is that people might actually see what we in the anti-vaccination world have been screaming from the rooftops for years, because some people just don't see things until they slap them right in the face and even then (as in this case) they remain permanently blinded.

The first post said:

"I was so relieved to get vaccinated for Covid-19 while I was pregnant this year, and to have some reassurance that I'm sharing my immune protections with my newborn now through breastfeeding. Happy to chat with expectant moms about questions if you're feeling hesitant."

Sadly the next post read as follows:

"Yesterday my littlest one passed away unexpectedly and suddenly at two and a half months. We don't have answers on how or why, but if you have little ones at home give them an extra squeeze today."

Update

Through doing a bit of chat-bombing on Plazma's channel on Odysee, I got him to read a bit of this article on his live show and then someone made a video of it. It's not a read aloud video but still pretty cool. Thanks to Lunac73. [76]

THE MOVEMENT WITH NO NAME

This is a post I wrote on Facebook that got shadow-banned in the thick of it. Wonder how it will fair now the truth is coming out?

The anti-vaccine movement is becoming a bit like Harry Potter and we are Voldemort or rather 'he who must not be named'. What is this angst about being called 'anti-vaccine'? Have we all turned into

---

[76] www.odysee.com/@lunac73:6/Interview-with-an-%E2%80%98Anti-Vaxxer%E2%80%99:5

millennials who must not be offended? Would you be offended if I called you anti-war? Anti-racism? Anti-cruelty? No?

The only people who should be afraid of the anti-vaccine label are doctors, nurses and bio-chemists for fear of losing their careers. This is the stance the VAXXED movement have chosen to take but where has it got them? Despite parroting the phrase over and over anyone who questions vaccines is automatically labelled with the awful curse of being an 'anti-vaxxer'. Oh the horror. Let's please not adopt the millennial cry of 'please do not say anything which shall offend ME'! We are grown-ups. Aren't we?

Some are taking up the name 'ex-vaxxers'. I just wonder why? Who are they trying to appease? Please sir, I don't mean to offend, I did try your way but it didn't agree with my disposition. Pur-lease. OK I get that some people are only just finding out about the horrors and lies of vaccines and they do not call themselves anti-vax because they don't even know if they ARE anti-vax yet, but WE (you know who you are) DO know. Not all of us know the WHOLE truth, some are lodged half way down the rabbit-hole sitting reading the supposedly 'scientific' studies where the holy grail of scientific truth will be found (hopefully one day) while some of us have seen the light at the end of the tunnel.

While we are all at various stages of our 'research' and it may take some time for the rest of you to join us for the party at the bottom of the rabbit hole can we please just stop with the pandering to the trolls and shills (who are obviously laughing their silly tits off at us all, but then that is what they do) and get on with fighting vaccines full on. None of this half-arsed, safer, spaced out nonsense. That is for newbies and also ultimately the vaccine market too. If you agree that vaccines are not safe and do not work then call yourself anti-vaccine and lets just get on with it because remember, sticks and stones may break your bones but vaccines can actually kill you!

"I speak now Harry Potter, directly to you. You have permitted your friends to die for you rather than face me yourself. I shall wait for one hour in the Forbidden Forest. If, at the end of that hour, you have not come to me, have not given yourself up, then battle recommences. This time, I shall enter the fray myself, Harry Potter, and I shall find you, and I shall punish every last man, woman, and child who has tried to conceal you from me. One hour." – J.K. Rowling, Harry Potter and the Deathly Hallows.

We ARE in the last hours of this battle and I am anti-vaccine and proud. We will not win this war by hiding in the shadows. If you are one of those stuck in the maze of scientific papers searching for the holy grail then stop for a moment and just research the 'germ theory' for one day. If you do not see the light at the end of the tunnel after that then carry on regardless. It will hit you eventually. In the meantime lets fight THEM and not each other and let's be honest about it. Lying is the pro-vaxxers game.

Are Va$$ines Legal?

I was doing a radio show and mentioned that I'd heard there was a law in 1840 which made inoculation illegal. The radio show host asked me for a source which I didn't have so went digging after the show to see what I could find. First stop Wiki (even though we know it's mostly bullshit) and their description of the 1840 Act…

"The 1840 Act

- **Made variolation illegal.**
- **Provided vaccination free of charge.**

In general, the disadvantages of variolation are the same as those of vaccination, but added to them is the general agreement that variolation was always more dangerous than vaccination." [77]

Indeed there was a law passed (an act, so a legal 'law' not a common law) and Wiki refers to it as a ban on 'variolation'. But in 1840 they weren't using 'variolation' which was a Chinese invention of blowing smallpox scabs up the nose (nice). That had long been replaced with 'inoculation' which was scratching smallpox pus into the skin of your victim instead of up the nose.

Wiki's description of variolation…

"Variolation was the method of inoculation first used to immunize individuals against smallpox (Variola) with material taken from a patient or a recently vaccinated individual, in the hope that a mild, but protective, infection would result.

The procedure was most commonly carried out by inserting/rubbing powdered smallpox scabs or fluid from pustules into superficial scratches made in the skin. The virus was normally spread through the air, infecting first the mouth,

---

[77] https://en.wikipedia.org/wiki/Vaccination_Act

nose, or respiratory tract, before spreading throughout the body via the lymphatic system."

Now Vaccines were 'invented' shortly before the ban and were basically the exact same procedure but instead of using pus from human smallpox spots they used pus from cows that had the pox, which they called cowpox for obvious reasons, although it's exactly the same thing really. So the only difference between this inoculation and vaccination was the cow element instead of another human. But they use humans in vaccination now too in the form of aborted fetuses.

Wiki's description of inoculation…

"Inoculation is a set of methods of artificially inducing immunity against various infectious diseases. The terms inoculation, vaccination and immunization are often used synonymously but there are some important differences among them."

They even admit the words are interchangeable. You'll rarely hear them use the inoculation word though for obvious reasons…I see a bit of legal shenanigans going on here. Why exactly did they make inoculation/variolation illegal anyway?

BECAUSE IT WAS KILLING PEOPLE THAT'S WHY.

Now how many other vaccines use cow pus to inoculate?

The answer is NONE yes. So as 'Vacca' means cow and vaccination was named after the cow element, none of the vaccines that came after could legally be called 'vacc'ines' at all. They are in fact INOCULATIONS which were the new variant of variolation which is to this day effectively BANNED.

"Why would they ban one form and not the other?" I hear you ask. Well anyone could make their own inoculation with a poxy person and a needle, simples. To do a vaccine though you would need to be a registered doctor or vaccinator AHA! Always follow the money.

Shortly after the ban 'VACC'inations' were made compulsory too!! KA'CHING! Now we just need a lawyer to look into this for us. I might be on to something? So if anyone wants to shove a 'vacc'ine into you, you can have them arrested, and so you jolly well should because they are still killing people. All we need now is a test case…

DR. JENNER AND THE MILKMAID

No this is not going to be a saucy story but while I have you here let's talk about that famous legend of how vaccines were discovered. I know we've all been sold the romantic story of a milkmaid schooling Jenner on the amazing science of 'immunity' but seriously if you believe that story I have a nice bridge to sell you. The whole concept of immunity (which we are told came from a lowly milkmaid) was in fact taken from the known concept of building immunity to poisons called Mithridatism. It had nothing to with germs or viruses unless you use the word virus in its original form which was 'poison'.

From Wiki: **Mithridatism. Not be confused with Mithraism.**

Mithridatism is the practice of protecting oneself against a poison by gradually self-administering non-lethal amounts. The word is derived from Mithridates VI the King of Pontus, who so feared being poisoned that he regularly ingested small doses, aiming to develop immunity.

Secondly, Jenner did not hear the tale from a milkmaid at all, he heard it from other natural philosophers of the time who had heard it from a farmer and not a milkmaid. This is stated in papers from the time. [78]

Inoculation was a common practice at this time, even Jenner himself had been inoculated for smallpox at school and had suffered with health issues from it into adulthood. This was why he looked for alternatives. I wonder if the farmers and milkmaids bragged of their 'immunity' to get out of having to be put through inoculation? Makes more sense to me than the official story.

So what IS this magical cowpox they claimed gave them immunity from smallpox?

Jenner's observations of 'cowpox' may have been grossly misinterpreted, as physicians, later on, discovered that cowpox pustules were only found on the udders of cows milked by filthy human hands and that cows roaming free in pastures were not affected by the disease.

So it was only a disease of dairy cows therefore it is the farming practices causing it and it is NOT contagious. Originally Jenner thought it had come from a horse complaint called 'horse grease'. This is also a disease of domestic working animals but let's look at the reason he thought this.

"In this dairy country a great number of cows are kept, and the office of milking is performed indiscriminately by men and maid servants. One of the former having been appointed to apply

[78] www.npr.org/sections/goatsandsoda/2018/02/01/582370199/whats-the-real-story-about-the-milkmaid-and-the-smallpox-vaccine

dressings to the heels of a horse affected with the grease, and not paying due attention to cleanliness, incautiously bears his part in milking the cows, with some particles of the infectious matter adhering to his fingers. When this is the case, it commonly happens that a disease is communicated to the cows, and from the cows to the dairymaids, which spreads through the farm until most of the cattle and domestics feel its unpleasant consequences. This disease has obtained the name of cow pox. It appears on the nipples of the cows in the form of irregular pustules." [79]

This story certainly makes it sound contagious doesn't it? But did anyone ask what the farmer dressed the horses heels with? I've tried to find an answer but can't, so maybe they would have used a similar remedy as for the cowpox seeing as they were interchangeable according to Jenner. Once the cows showed symptoms they already had a treatment which was deemed to work so it must have been used extensively. These two treatments consisted of Vitriolum Cupri and Vitriolum Zinci. Seeing as no-one seems to ask the question 'could it be the noxious treatments causing the pustules/blisters?' I looked up these common treatment ingredients liberally slathered all over dairy cows teats. [80] [81] [82] [83]

Vitriolum cupri
Formula: $CuSO_4 \cdot 5H_2O$
Latin synonym of: Chalcanthite

Look up Chalcanthite and this is what it says about the **health risks: Hazardous in case of skin contact (irritant), of eye contact (irritant), of ingestion, of inhalation. Acute oral toxicity (LD50): 300mg/kg [Rat.].**

Vitriolum Zinci album nativum
Formula: $ZnSO_4 \cdot 7H_2O$
Latin synonym of: Goslarite

---

[79] www.viroliegy.com/2022/02/03/edward-jenners-smallpox-paper-1798/

[80] www.mindat.org/show.php?id=4929&ld

[81] www.mindat.org/min-959.html

[82] www.mindat.org/min-4546.html

[83] www.mindat.org/min-1731.html

So the maids would be getting this toxic skin irritant on their hands and then spreading it from cow to cow but also some of it must have gotten into the milk. So there is your 'viral contagion' of spreading poison skin to skin and even possibly being ingested in the milk.

Now to my next point which recently came up from the Weston Price camp that drinking 'raw' milk could have been the reason for the milkmaids 'immunity' to smallpox, which I've already established is a lie but need to clear this fallacy up too.

Milkmaids no doubt did drink raw milk but so did everyone in those days as Pasteur and pasteurization did not come about for another 100 years at least. There are many other factors which would have made milkmaids and other country folk healthier.

Fresh air, clean fresh water, fruit and veg fresh unadulterated from nature, regular income and generally a higher standard of living than town or city dwellers of the same social status.

There was an excellent (although germ theory laden) short documentary on the horrific treatment of foodstuffs in Victorian days on YouTube (but it's disappeared now). A few years later indeed but frankly it can only have been worse in the 18th century. If you thought Victorians had a healthier diet, think again. It was mentioned that they added borax to old milk to cover the sour taste. Makes you wonder what they added in Jenner's time before sending the milk to market without refrigeration, apart from the contamination of 'treatments' for blistered cow nipples.

In the documentary they end up blaming the deaths of children on bacteria (TB) in the milk though and sideline any chemical cause of death as usual. This was what prompted the need for the pasteurization process.

Nice bit of circular reasoning and scapegoating again. The original claim of immunity in the case of cowpox was never even proven. Milk maids and other people who regularly milked cows could get it over and over again. So if they weren't immune to the cowpox how on earth did that translate to an immunity to smallpox?

EDWARD JENNER

"Even Dr. Major Greenwood, Chief Statistician to the Ministry of Health, declared in 1929 that: "In Jenner's classical paper no mistake was omitted that could have possibly been made, and there was a good deal of evidence that Jenner had been a rogue." In his well-known work 'Epidemics and Crowd Diseases' (1935),

Professor Greenwood wrote: "Most of Jenner's time during the last twenty years of his life was spent in attempting the impossible, i.e., in attempting to convince his correspondents that no properly cowpoxed person could get smallpox."
– M. Beddow Bayly M.R.C.S., L.R.C.P (1936)

So back to my main points for writing this – immunity is another fairytale concept. Toxic treatments and other pollutants were the causes of smallpox (and cowpox). Jenner was a fraudster or just a deluded do-gooder. A milkmaid did not invent the 'immune system'. Raw milk is not a human superfood, it is meant for baby cows.

DIAGNOSIS LIE

"During the last considerable epidemic at the turn of the century, I was a member of the Health Committee of London Borough Council, and I learned how the credit of vaccination is kept statistically by diagnosing all the revaccinated cases (of smallpox) as pustular eczema, varioloid or what not...except smallpox."
– George Bernard Shaw (1906)

Smallpox itself was never eradicated either, it seems they did the old name-swap on it just like they did with polio and many other diseases to follow.

Sounds familiar huh?

It also should be noted that the worst smallpox 'epidemics' happened AFTER the vaccines had been liberally enforced.

Nice work Jenner.

POLIO

ALS AND THE ICE BUCKET CHALLENGE
(OR, WHATEVER HAPPENED TO POLIO?)

OK a bunch of celebs throwing buckets of ice over their heads and bragging who their other famous friends are, to raise money for 'medical research' which will include millions of animals being tortured for a bogus cure for something which was and is being caused by the very people who will be benefitting from those funds is just making my blood boil. So here are some facts:

ALS or AMYOTROPHIC LATERAL SCLEROSIS or Lou Gehrig's Disease cannot be differentiated significantly from Post-Polio Syndrome or Chronic Polio. Polio has supposedly been eradicated by vaccines. Vaccines are a multi-billion dollar business which if caught out would cause the demise of Big pHarma. If word got out that polio was in fact NOT eradicated but in fact 'spreading' like wild-fire under various names, OOPS!

Diseases with varying degrees of the same symptoms as polio and falling under the umbrella of Motor Neuron disease:

- Amyotrophic Lateral Sclerosis (Als) Or Lou Gehrig's Disease
- Guillain-Barré Syndrome
- Myasthenia Gravis
- MS
- Acute Flaccid Paralysis (AFP)
- Transverse Myelitis
- Viral or Aseptic Meningitis
- Chinese Paralytic Syndrome
- Chronic Fatigue Syndrome
- Epidemic Cholera
- Cholera Morbus
- Spinal Meningitis
- Spinal Apoplexy
- Inhibitory Palsy
- Intermittent Fever
- Famine Fever
- Worm Fever

- Bilious Remittent Fever
- Ergotism
- ME
- Post-Polio Syndrome

"Polio has not been eradicated at all. And will not be eradicated. Polio has been renamed ... why have Acute Flaccid Paralysis and Polio been put together? Because Acute Flaccid Paralysis is a catch-all name for what looks like polio, and what you call polio when the crucial polio viral tests don't show polio VIRUSES at all. ...While the cases of 'polio' have gone down, cases of polio which didn't return a positive virus test, and which are now called 'Acute Flaccid Paralysis' have skyrocketed. Nice little bit of magicians' sleight of hand...???! A parent who saw that WHO website page, wouldn't know that Acute Flaccid Paralysis was simply polio of old, which covered the same syndromes and symptoms, caused by a large variety of viruses, as well as various toxins. A parent looking at the WHO website, would think to themselves, 'Acute Flaccid Paralysis' must be some other 'valid' disease in its own right...

All the kids who used to be on clumsy iron lungs, are now on high tech iron lungs and renamed under the autoimmune moniker called Transverse Myelitis and no doubt other creative titles to spread the decoys around. And here is your proof. Hidden away in the forward of a book, by a specialist doctor. Of course, paralysed cases of transverse myelitis on modern iron lungs isn't something either the media, or WHO will shout from the rooftops. So today, instead of kids with polio in callipers and iron lungs, we have lots of kids with autoimmunity, and ... widespread chronic diseases. In 1958 (the year mass polio vaccination was rolled out in the USA) the CDC formally adopted the 'Best available paralytic Poliomyelitis case count' or BAPPCC:

Cases must be clinically and epidemiologically compatible with Poliomyelitis, must have resulted in paralysis and must have a residual neurological deficit 60 days after onset of initial symptoms ... the BAPPCC does not include cases of nonparalytic Poliomyelitis, of those in which paralysis is more transient. The original purpose of developing these criteria was to omit cases possibly due to enteroviruses other than Polioviruses."

– Polio and Lemmings by Hilary Butler (May 2011)

People who showed polio like symptoms that previously would have been diagnosed as polio were now being diagnosed as:

- Acute Flaccid Paralysis (AFP)
- Transverse Myelitis
- Viral or Aseptic Meningitis
- Guillain-Barré Syndrome (GBS)
- Chinese Paralytic Syndrome
- Chronic Fatigue Syndrome
- Epidemic Cholera
- Cholera Morbus
- Spinal Meningitis
- Spinal Apoplexy
- Inhibitory Palsy
- Intermittent Fever
- Famine Fever
- Worm Fever
- Bilious Remittent Fever
- Ergotis
- ME
- Post-Polio Syndrome aka GBS

Coxsackie virus and echo viruses can cause paralytic syndromes that are clinically indistinguishable from paralytic Poliomyelitis.

SO polio didn't go away, it was 'renamed'!! (and they're still doing it!) CLEVER DICKS. SO…where did polio originally come from?

Originally it was pesticides like DDT. Some of the first outbreaks correlate with crop spraying with toxic pesticides.

Milk! Polio outbreaks were linked to milk with high pesticide levels and more recently raw milk.

Next we have vaccines. Some polio outbreaks correlate with mass BCG and DTP vaccine drives.

Parents should also know some of the same chemicals used to spray pesticides (Tween 20, Tween 80, Triton X-100, Nonoxyenol-9) are still present in childhood vaccines.

The common denominator in all these is pesticides.

Now we have ALS and the Ice Bucket Challenge which has already raised over $500,000,000. What's the betting they are looking for yet another vaccine for the exact same disease they were supposed to have already eradicated and on which the whole vaccine industry pivots?

OH THE IRONY!!!

AND consider this – they were already trying this ploy in 2019 just before covid, so it had been predicted (PLANNED) already but obviously stalled.

Read this old news article from July 2019 and join the dots (I've joined most of them for you).

This important news article from the *New York Daily News* has been censored from EU countries so I have had to post it here from private messages sent to me. [84]

My comments are in brackets throughout.

The CDC issued a vital signs warning Tuesday as it prepares for a potential outbreak of the 'polio-like' illness Acute Flaccid Myelitis (AFM) in the fall. Since 2014, AFM has struck children in increasing numbers from August to October with peak outbreaks occurring on even-numbered years. Although doctors have linked a number of cases in the initial 2014 outbreak to enterovirus D-68, health officials have not yet been able to determine the exact cause of the illness that has caused many children to become paralyzed.

(In other words they have no clue as to the cause)

Ahead of the outbreaks, the CDC issued a warning on Tuesday including information on AFM and what doctors should do if cases are suspected. Although rare, the illness is serious, doctors have warned. "Improving the understanding of AFM is a public health priority. The overall rarity of this condition and absence of a confirmatory test highlight the need for increased vigilance among providers seeing pediatric patients with acute onset of flaccid limb weakness in the late summer and fall".

(If they have no test for this, ergo they have no test for polio either, so what is the difference?)

"Ongoing national AFM surveillance will provide an important bridge between research and public health response and will be critical for the development of optimal treatment and prevention recommendations," the CDC warned.

Children often have symptoms of an upper respiratory infection,

---

[84] https://www.nydailynews.com/news/national/ny-cdc-vital-warning-outbreak-polio-afm-20190709-kllyufok7nbk7c346xv5pu6fx4-story.html

and children may later have difficulty breathing and 'flaccid weakness' that develops into paralysis where they are unable to move their limbs. Although 2019 is not likely to be a peak year as previous peak outbreaks have occurred on even-number years, the CDC is preparing as August to October are when the most outbreaks are seen from year-to-year.

(Same months as 'polio' outbreaks)

The CDC urged that testing protocol from doctors in suspected patients is crucial to helping determine the cause of the condition and refining the definition. "Prompt recognition, early specimen collection, and reporting of all suspected cases to public health are important goals for AFM national surveillance," the CDC said. They also said that despite testing patients for a variety of pathogens only 3% of cerebral spinal fluid (CSF) specimens yielded a result in 2018. This data suggests routine enterovirus, rhinovirus or PCR testing of CSF are "unlikely to confirm the cause of these outbreaks."

(These tests are bullshit)

"Early recognition and specimen collection from suspected AFM patients are essential to optimizing pathogen detection and determining whether single or multiple etiologies are responsible for the recent outbreaks," the CDC states.

Dr. Benjamin Greenberg, a neurologist at the UT Southwestern and Children's Health in Dallas, previously told the Daily News that if AFM is caused by an enterovirus like D-68, the viruses could be detected by swabs at the back of the throat because that is where they replicate – not from CSF samples or stool samples like the polio virus.

"Although 44% of confirmed AFM cases in 2018 had an enterovirus or rhinovirus identified in respiratory specimens, approximately half were negative," the CDC said.

(If half do not have the 'virus' then the 'virus' cannot be the cause)

The CDC states that timeliness is essential for testing these viruses, because they may have a short time frame when they are detectable — meaning some viruses may not have been detected due to the timeliness of testing despite increased protocol.

(More bullshit. Explain this 'timeframe' for detecting 'viruses')

This could be the key to determining the cause of the illness, and potentially developing a vaccine, doctors have said.

(So they want to develop ANOTHER polio vaccine for a disease that they supposedly eradicated with vaccines?)

Patients with suspected cases of AFM should undergo immediate testing, and doctors should report cases quickly to health departments and the CDC, the health agency said. "In the absence of a confirmatory diagnostic test for AFM, management decisions for individual patients in the acute setting should be informed by careful review of the patient's signs and symptoms, laboratory testing, MRI results, and other test results, including electromyography, and in close consultation with infectious disease specialists and neurologists," the CDC stated in its vital signs warning. "To provide additional specificity for reporting of patients with suspected AFM to health departments, the Council of State and Territorial Epidemiologists modified the clinical criteria for reporting of patients suspected of AFM in June 2019 to include MRI evidence of spinal lesions with at least some gray matter involvement, in addition to acute flaccid limb weakness."

(Just like they modified the criteria for polio diagnosis after the vaccine was rolled out)

In 2018, the nation saw its largest outbreak of AFM, with 233 confirmed cases.

(That is more than the original polio outbreaks!!)

Nine cases have been confirmed already this year, with health officials prepping around the world for a possible increase in cases in the coming fall months.

(I'll bet, prepping for damage control of people cottoning on to their bullshit cover-up of the continuing polio outbreaks)

At this point I've come across a nice bit of historical data which I'll add here for your further research into this very long running scam/cover-up…

LET'S TAKE A LOOK AT HISTORY AND POLIO!

(Thank you Caitlin for this quick, yet extremely important history lesson).

1824: Metal workers had suffered for centuries from a paralysis similar to polio caused by the lead and arsenic in the metals they were working with. English scientist John Cooke observed: 'The fumes from these metals, or the receptance of them in solution into the stomach, often causes paralysis'.

1890: Lead arsenate pesticide started to be sprayed in the US up to 12 times every summer to kill codling moth on apple crops.

1892: Polio outbreaks began to occur in Vermont, an apple growing region. In his report the Government Inspector Dr. Charles Caverly noted that parents reported that some children fell ill after eating fruit. He stated that 'infantile paralysis' usually occurred in families with more than one child, and as no efforts were made at isolation it was very certain it was non-contagious' (with only one child in the family having been struck).

1907: Calcium arsenate comes into use primarily on cotton crops.

1908: In a Massachusetts town with three cotton mills and apple orchards, 69 children suddenly fell ill with infantile paralysis.

1909: The UK bans apple imports from the States because of heavy lead arsenate residues.

1921: Franklin D. Roosevelt develops polio after swimming in Bay of Fundy, New Brunswick. Toxicity of water may have been due to pollution run-off.

1943: DDT is introduced, a neurotoxic pesticide. Over the next several years it comes into widespread use in American households. For example, wall paper impregnated with DDT was placed in children's bedrooms.

1943: A polio epidemic in the UK town of Broadstairs, Kent is linked to a local dairy where cows were washed down with DDT.

1944: Albert Sabin reports that a major cause of sickness and death of American troops based in the Philippines was Poliomyelitis. US military camps there were sprayed daily with DDT to kill mosquitoes. Neighboring Philippine settlements were not affected.

1944: NIH reports that DDT damages the same anterior horn cells that are damaged in infantile paralysis.

1946: Gebhaedt shows polio seasonality correlates with fruit harvest.

1949: Endocrinologist Dr. Morton Biskind, a practitioner and medical researcher, found that DDT causes 'lesions in the spinal cord similar to human polio'.

1950: US Public Health Industrial Hygiene Medical Director, J.G. Townsend, notes the similarity between parathion poisoning and polio and believes that some polio might be caused by eating fruits or vegetables with parathion residues.

1951: Dr. Biskind treats his polio patients as poisoning victims, removing toxins from food and environment, especially DDT contaminated milk and butter. Dr. Biskind writes: "Although young animals are more susceptible to the effects of DDT than adults, so far as the available literature is concerned, it does not appear that the effects of such concentrations on infants and children have even been considered".

1949-1951: Other doctors report they are having success treating polio with anti-toxins used to treat poisoning, dimercaprol and ascorbic acid. Example: Dr. F. R. Klenner reported: "In the Poliomyelitis epidemic in North Carolina in 1948 60 cases of this disease came under our care… The treatment was massive doses of vitamin C every two to four hours. Children up to four years received vitamin C injection intramuscularly…all patients were clinically well after 72 hours".

1950: Dr. Biskind presents evidence to the US Congress that pesticides were the major cause of polio epidemics. He is joined by Dr. Ralph Scobey who reported he found clear evidence of poisoning when analyzing chemical traces in the blood of polio victims. Comment: This was a no-no. The viral causation theory was not something to be questioned. The careers of prominent virologists and health authorities were threatened. Biskind and Scobey's ideas were subjected to ridicule.

1953: Clothes are moth-proofed by washing them in EQ-53, a formula containing DDT.

1953: Dr. Biskind writes: "It was known by 1945 that DDT was stored in the body fat of mammals and appears in their milk…yet far from admitting a causal relationship between DDT and polio that is so obvious, which in any other field of biology would be instantly accepted, virtually the entire apparatus of communication, lay and scientific alike, has been devoted to denying, concealing, suppressing, distorting and attempts to convert into its opposite this overwhelming evidence. Libel, slander, and economic boycott have not been overlooked in this campaign".

1954: Legislation recognizing the dangers of persistent pesticides is enacted, and a phase out of DDT in the US accelerates along with a shift of sales of DDT to third world countries (note that DDT is phased out at the same time as widespread polio vaccinations begin). Saying that, polio cases sky rocket only in communities that accept the polio vaccine, as the polio vaccine is laced with heavy metals and other toxins, so the paralysis narrative starts all over again. As the polio vaccines cause huge spikes in polio, the misinformed public demand more polio vaccine and the cycle spirals skyward exponentially.

1956: The American Medical Association mandated that all licensed medical doctors could no longer classify polio as polio. All polio diagnosis would be rejected in favor of Guillain-Barre Syndrome, AFP (acute flaccid paralysis), Bell's Palsy, Cerebral Palsy, ALS, (Lou-Gehrig's Disease), MS, MD etc. etc. This sleight of hand was fabricated with the sole intent of giving the public the impression that the polio vaccine was successful at decreasing polio or eradicating polio. The public bought this hook, line and sinker and to this very day, many pro vaccine arguments are ignited by the manufactured lie regarding the polio vaccine eradicating polio.

1962: Rachel Carson's Silent Spring is published.

1968: DDT registration cancelled for the US.

2008: Acute Flaccid Paralysis (AFP) is still raging in many parts of the world where pesticide use is high, and DDT is still used. AFP. MS, MD, Bell's Palsy, cerebral palsy, ALS (Lou Gehrig's Disease), Guillain-Barre are all catch basket diagnosis, all similar in symptoms, tied to heavy metal poisoning and high toxic load.

2008: WHO states on its website: 'There is no cure for polio. Its effects are irreversible'. Conclusion: modern belief that polio is caused by a virus is an ongoing tragedy for the children of the world. Public funds are wasted on useless and dangerous vaccines when the children could be treated with antitoxins. A call into failing vaccine mythology is warranted, as is a complete investigation of the real agenda being executed against humanity involving science, chemicals, vaccines, the medical field in general, and the government.

I heard on UK Column News that this same thing is being pushed in the UK, particularly in the area I used to live. They claim to have found 'polio' in the waste water and are going to be pushing the IPV on children aged 1 to 9 in the UK.

So this thing is not a flash in the pan. [85]

Why are the media and CDC suddenly screaming about polio cases in wastewater but not human cases? What is causing outbreaks in New York if it has been supposedly eradicated?

THE POLIO VACCINES THEMSELVES

This will run contrary to *everything* you have been taught by those propping up pharmaceutical companies, and has even been *omitted* by the media outlets reporting on it, but the CDC were forced to admit the polio virus in the wastewater was *vaccine-derived*. [86]

(I have an archived back up from the Waybackmachine in case they try to delete the evidence).

"UPDATE – Vaccine-Derived Poliovirus: In July 2022, CDC was notified of a case of polio caused by vaccine-derived poliovirus

---

[85] UK Column News (scroll to about 19 mins in)

[86] https://www.cdc.gov/vaccines/vpd/polio/hcp/vaccine-derived-poliovirus-faq.html

type 2 (VDPV2) in an unvaccinated individual from Rockland County, New York, and is consulting with the New York State Department of Health on their investigation. Public health experts are working to understand how and where the individual was infected and provide protective measures, such as vaccination services to the community to prevent the spread of polio to under and unvaccinated individuals."

Now you need to watch out for cognitive dissonance, but they admit the wastewater polio is 'vaccine-derived', as in…the polio vaccines themselves are causing the outbreak.

POLIO IS NOT CONTAGIOUS

Look especially at point 10. This is one of the biggest cover ups ever!

14 Things You Didn't Know About Polio

1. A pesticide common in the 1800's was called Paris Green. A green liquid because it was a combination of copper and arsenic or lead and arsenic. Some of the most toxic substances known to humankind.

2. This pesticide worked by causing neurological damage in the bugs, causing organ failure.

3. Polio consists of symptoms synonymous with neurological damage, causing organ failure.

4. Heavy metal poisoning from lead, mercury and other similar heavy metals manifest lesions on neurological tissues, meaning the toxin destroys the nerve/communication pathways connecting the brain to the organs in the body. (Check out 'Mercury Poisoning – The Minamata Story' on YouTube).

5. Polio victims present lesions on neurological tissue, that cause the organs to malfunction all around the body. (lungs, heart, nerves that control walking etc.).

6. Polio outbreaks hit throughout the summer, only during pesticide spraying times. (not the sunless and damp winter/spring seasons regarding other disease outbreaks).

7. Polio had and has NO ability to spread from infected victims to the uninfected. Polio infected clusters of people in the exact same areas, suddenly and swiftly.

8. Parents report finding their children paralyzed in and around apple orchards. One of the most heavily pesticide sprayed crops of the time (with lead arsenate or copper arsenate) were apple orchards.

9. President Roosevelt became paralyzed overnight while on his farm in the summer, which contained many crops, including apple orchards. He also swam the day prior in a bay that was heavily polluted by industrial agricultural run-off.

10. Dr. Ralph Scobey and Dr. Mortind Biskind testified in front of the U.S. Congress in 1951 that the paralysis around the country known as polio was being caused by industrial poisons and that a virus theory was purposely fabricated by the chemical industry and the government to deflect litigation away from both parties.

11. In 1956 the AMA (The American Medical Association) instructed each licensed medical doctor that they could no longer classify polio as polio, or their license to practice would be terminated. Any paralysis was now to be diagnosed as AFP (acute flaccid paralysis) MS, MD, Bell's Palsy, Cerebral Palsy, ALS (Lou Gehrig's Disease), Guillain-Barré, Meningitis etc. This was orchestrated purposely to make the public believe Polio was eradicated by the polio vaccine campaign but because the polio vaccine contained toxic ingredients directly linked to paralysis, polio cases (not identified as polio) were skyrocketing...but only in vaccinated areas. The first polio vaccine was worked on by Dr. Jonas Salk and human experiments using this vaccine were conducted purposely on orphans in government/church run institutions because they were vulnerable and didn't require any parental consent signatures, as they had no parents. The vaccine was 'declared safe' by 'medicine' (as they always are even though that vaccine was killing and paralyzing monkeys in test trials) and that vaccine gave 40,000 orphans polio, permanently paralyzed hundreds and killed at least 10 children. All injuries and deaths under reported of course by the same authorities who orchestrated the atrocity. This was called The Cutter Incident. A focused attack on defenseless children, by people charged with their care. A poisoning of innocent children and then the excuses and apologies, regarding how it won't happen again. Is this pattern still occurring today?

12. **(deleted as contained spurious dis-info about 'cancer viruses' and 'AIDS viruses' which have never been proven to exist). SV40 is monkey cell debris, animal and human cell debris is in EVERY vaccine.**

13. In the book Virus Mania by Torsten Engelbrecht and Claus Köhnlein, top scientists in the field declare that polio doesn't and has never qualified as a viral disease because it fails to spread from person to person or animal to animal. If it's not a viral disease, then what is it? The answer is heavy metal and other forms of toxic poisoning that causes partial or full paralysis (destruction of the nervous system). Join the dots.

14. When someone talks of any disease, in this day and age, they're often just repeating what they were told by the government. When someone today repeats anything about polio and polio elimination based on vaccination, they're repeating known lies, told by known liars. Repeating what you're told and intelligence aren't the same thing. Repeating or intelligence. The choice is yours. Repeaters are FIRM IN THEIR BELIEFS yet have NEVER researched beyond what they were told to believe. Such firm belief, with ZERO RESEARCH, is illogical and irrational.

Research the hidden history of polio, the disease that never was, at westonaprice.org 'Pesticides and Polio A Critique of Scientific Literature'. Further research regarding the polio deception can be found in these books: 'Health and Nutrition Secrets That Can Save Your Life' by Dr. Russell Blaylock and 'Official Stories: Counter-Arguments for a Culture in Need' by Liam Scheff.

POLIO WAS NEVER 'ERADICATED'

This is a post from Kathleen Berrett, the mother of a victim of modern day 'polio', written in 2018.

"Seven heart breaking years ago my perfectly healthy son became a ventilator dependent quadriplegic due to the vaccine Gardasil. Whether you call the condition TM or AFM they are both terms for polio renamed. Colton fought so hard to get better. He was so strong and pushed himself trying to achieve a normal body that he once had never to achieve it in this lifetime. Gardasil took his happy life from him. Gardasil took everything away from him that you take for granted like breathing, being able to walk, scratching your own itch, hugging someone, dressing yourself. Gardasil took my son from me. Merck knows these risks exist. The Government knows these risks exist. Doctors know these risks exist yet they still administer vaccines because of money! They aren't administering vaccines for your health and safety, it's all about money! There's no true safety studies on vaccines; CDC destroys the info showing bad side effects from vaccines. Please do your research. I did mine too late. My son is gone! I miss him like crazy. You can protect your kids, don't be a fool… don't trust a doctor that makes money pushing vaccines.

READ A TRUE VACCINE INSERT. DARE YOUR DOCTOR TO READ THE VACCINE INSERT. WHAT ARE THE INGREDIENTS? NEUROTOXINS!

I miss you son."

Just so you know Colton didn't die from the effects of a jab, he took his own life because the life he had was no longer worth living. Sure modern medicine could have kept him 'alive' for as long as he wanted. What they took from him was health and quality of life. No meds could bring that back. RIP Colton.

Colton's story is in the book 'The HPV Vaccine On Trial: Seeking Justice for a Generation Betrayed' by Mary Holland. His story is also highlighted in 'Vaxxed 2 The People's Truth' on Peeps TV through Roku and at www.vaxxed2.com.

POLIO IS BACK

Sounds like the title of a cheesy romcom B movie doesn't it? Sadly it's not though, it's just those pesky fear-mongerers again, up to their old tricks.

The irony is though, for the last 30 years or so all the pro-vaxxers have been selling their dodgy wares with the favourite tagline 'vaccines eradicated polio'. (Get your damned vaccines). Literally that was their whole selling point, so what now? Are they saying that was a big fat lie? Eradicated isn't like an injunction and the virus snuck in the back door and grabbed you. Eradicated means gone. Poof.

New York is one of the most vaccinated states in the US – hell they even mandated some of them and tried to force the Jewish community to get all theirs too in 2019. They didn't even need to force the polio vax on anyone though, even most anti-vaxxers have had that one even if they don't know it.

When I was a nipper back in the 1960's we all got a sugar cube. One sugar cube laced with God knows what and that was it. Done. Obviously you can't give that to a baby and I have a vague memory of it, so probably around 5 years old.

When it was time for my kids in the 1980's the polio was no longer given on a sugar cube, it was nestled in a 3-in-1 needle shot called DTP (for diphtheria, polio and tetanus). Now they wanted to give that to my 2 month old baby!

I often wondered what the motivation was for all these new combined vaccines. The official narrative is that it means less jabs. That is a lie though as they just give fewer jabs more often which still adds up to MORE jabs.

Single jabs are easier to blame for immediate and obvious effects so could it be that when a particular jab gets some bad rap and becomes less marketable they just sneak it in next to the perceived essential jabs making it impossible to discern which poison is causing which 'side effects'? That makes more sense.

Did you know now you can no longer get a tetanus jab? It is no longer available so when you think you're getting a tetanus jab you are actually getting 3 jabs. DTP in the UK but now changed again to DTaP and Tdap. Who knows what shite they're palming off on you instead of cleaning your wounds properly?

Today the polio 'jab' is nestled in a SIX in one jab called the Hexavalent. Along with it is the very suspiciously added HepB. But before that there was another 6-in-1 called 'Hexavac' and another called 'Infanrix' which were quietly 'discontinued' by the European Union with a lame excuse of 'waning immunity' of the HepB faction in it. [87]

BUT if you dig a little deeper the story is much darker. As usual. There were DEATHS involved. Admittedly only a few definitively pointed to the vaccines but as we now know those few were just the tip of an iceberg which marketing-wise could sink their Titanic. [88]

It's also a patent issue, when a new vaccine is patented that means maximum profits for the patent holder (the vaccine developer). When the patent runs out the vaccine is no longer profitable so why not mix it in with other no longer profitable vaccines to make a new combo which they can also patent. The single shot then becomes 'unavailable' because no-one wants to provide unprofitable drugs. So much for vaccine producers being saints, working for free to save humanity. That is utter bullshit and pure marketing sloganism. Vaccines are ALL about the money!!

Let's take measles as an example. Back in the 1960's again measles was no big deal. Apparently it was said EVERYONE got it. It was seen

---

[87] www.ema.europa.eu/en/medicines/human/EPAR/hexavac
[88] www.arzneitelegramm.de/journal/j0305_a.php3

as a rite of passage in a way. No-one was scared of it, in fact people used to actively try to induce it with measles parties to 'get it over with'. I myself allegedly had 'GERMAN measles' which they claim is a separate disease but the only difference for a clinical diagnosis was the spots were a 'little less red'. Clearly it is the same thing and despite measles being said to be the most contagious disease we know of, no-one in my family but me got it.

So marketing a measles vaccine was always going to be hard work but they tried anyway. The effects of the first vaccine though were MUCH worse than actual measles. [89]

So they tweaked it a couple of times but by then measles had virtually disappeared on its own and their vaccine was just not selling. They tried mandates for school attendance in some USA states but it never was a success financially. So then they decided to invent the MMR. Combining 3 failed (and surely outdated patents) vaccines into one big marketing ploy.

Along came Dr Andrew Wakefield to throw a spanner in their dastardly plot. NOT an anti-vaccine man, just an anti-combined vaccine man. He naively thought that splitting the 3 vaccines apart would solve the problem he had uncovered of the MMR possibly causing gut problems in Autistic children. In his naivety he didn't realise he was asking vaccine companies to give away their old, no longer patented vaccines, for free. Silly man.

This process of new vaccines, failure and/or damage, patents running out, recombining the same ingredients to produce new marketable products has been going on since the 60's.

If these miraculous concoctions were responsible for 'eradicating' all these deadly (so we're told) diseases successfully then why do they always get shelved? I think you should now get the idea why…

So now back to this new polio 'outbreak' in New York. Is it really an outbreak? It seems it's an outbreak of 'polio in the poop' to be frank.

So NO it's NOT a polio outbreak, an outbreak of bullshit (or rather humanshit) from local ex-spurts is what it is. No doubt another testdemic using the old PCR to detect in silico combinations of RNA which means absolutely NOTHING in bodily fluids let alone the sewage works! Except possibly some new sales pitch for general vaccines (not covid tech/gen shots) which have been waning because

---

[89] Why It Took So Long to Eliminate Measles
www.history.com/news/measles-vaccine-disease

of us all being locked down for a year.

Some of us knew all along that polio wasn't caused by any virus, that it was caused by various pesticides, starting with the old arsenic sprayed on orchards then DDT sprayed on everything including kids in swimming pools, even while eating their dinner!!

We also knew it never went away – they just pretended it did by diagnosing the exact same symptoms as anything but polio.

So how can it be back? What could they possibly gain by dusting off that old chestnut? As they seem to be inventing new reasons for all the symptoms people are having after the con-vid jabs it must be that. We know there are symptoms of paralysis coming out. Strokes are a kind of paralysis, Guillain Barré is another name for polio, as is Bell's Palsy, both quite popular lately.

Are there plans, or have they already started spraying new noxious chemicals in cities like they've been doing in China?

Are they pre-empting the known side-effects of future spraying? Or is it just the jabs? A combination of both, covering all bases probably.

So before you all rush out to get your 'polio boosters' maybe have a little think about this – an article I wrote in 2014, all about the polio lie.

I promise it won't hurt, you may even find it helpful.

NEW 'MYSTERY' ILLNESSES – HERE COMES COVAIDS

I can't believe I have to do this and if you've already read and understood my articles on germ theory, virus theory and contagion then you probably don't need to read this but as it is not going away I feel it has to be addressed. It could be something, or it could be nothing. It could be another shot over the boughs or it could be just a fishing expedition. The person who sent me this seemed to think it was a distraction or a cover story. What am I talking about?

THIS (from The Sun newspaper, Feb 2022): [90]

"BRITS have been urged to come forward for HIV tests after heterosexual diagnoses of the illness have overtaken those in gay men. It's the first time the cases have shifted in decades and research shows that testing rates have dropped a third."

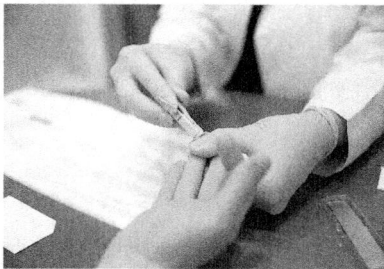

First off we need to ask some obvious questions.

1. How did an allegedly 'sexually transmitted disease' get transmitted during the height of lockdowns when all chances of sexually active people encountering each other's body parts were quashed? No pubs, clubs, gigs, parties. No hugging, kissing not even shaking of hands let alone bumping of sexual parts was allowed.

2. How did all these randy people get HIV tested when no-one could even get past hospital/hellth clinic security even to see their dying mum? This is so blatantly a lie, either the media and whoever fed them this story are morons OR they believe their readers are morons with the memories of goldfish. (Actually the goldfish memory thing has even been debunked now. They may actually have better memories than Sun readers to be fair.)

As if the lie is not obvious enough they even put their 'not so secret

---

anymore) calling card to this piece of blatant propaganda.
test and know their HIV status.

During 2020 heterosexuals testing for HIV dropped by 33 per cent, compared to just seven per cent in gay and bisexual men.

Oh and I almost forgot another side note (literally it's at the side of the original Sun article right next to the secret number in fact).

Headline from the Sun: **MUM'S LEGACY Harry breaks silence after Camilla news to vow to finish mum Diana's HIV work**

Yup it looks like they are going to go with this one with 'Royal' stamp of approval. They really don't want us breeding, that is patently obvious .[91]

> So people who have experimented with drugs that require injecting with a needle now need an HIV test.

(Facebook post from Deborah Harris)

You know what I think? I think they've plateaued with their mRNA covid shot campaign, in fact it's fallen over the cliff of the plateau and is now skydiving. There is now an orderly queue of other pHarma businesses waiting to cash in on the back of this money laundering operation and maybe the AIDS business is next in line. People are not afraid of that old covid virus anymore, but maybe they would be afraid of the old bogeyman that's been simmering away in the gay closet since the 80's. Maybe they're hoping to inject some new life into the old dog yet?

OR maybe it's just another marketing ploy for GUESS WHAT?

Yeh you guessed it, ANOTHER VACCINE!

Now don't you think it's strange that in all this time they've never come up with a vaccine until now? Apparently they were testing one in Africa last year. [92]

The results were as usual nothing short of disastrous but no doubt that won't stop them, it never did before. So are we about to see another rollout of a new gene-therapy shot cunningly disguised as

---

[91] www.thesun.co.uk/fabulous/17605741/prince-harry-continue-diana-work-hiv/

[92] www.sciencenews.org/article/aids-hiv-vaccine-anniversary-immunity-antibodies

another new 'vaccine'? Perfect timing or what? (Yes that is sarcasm indeed).

The links to the old AIDS fiasco were pretty clear from the start to some of us, even the major league players were the same.

1. Fauci and his deadly drug AZT for AIDS and now his new deadly drug Remdesivir for covid. An 'anti-viral' drug which branched out from the AIDS industry as did all other 'anti-virals'.

2. Kary Mullis and his PCR lab tool (stop calling it a test) which he clearly came out at the time to expose its use as fraudulent for testing for the HI virus. (Coincidence that he died shortly before the curtains opened on the covid show?).

Another parallel was the 'behind the scenes' battle about the isolation of the actual virus. They never did prove its existence, never isolated anything, and Deusberg seemed to be the only dissident voice asking for proof it caused the made-up disease they were calling AIDS which was clearly caused by a cocktail of illegal and legal medical drugs.

It was the whole HIV/AIDS debacle that sparked the 'do viruses even exist?' movement which has grown even bigger through this covid scam so why would they risk linking the two together again now? Are they really stupid or do they think WE are stupid? Are they hoping it's all forgotten as we are a couple of generations past that PLUS they've managed to kill off a large portion of the generation that lived through it?

If like some you believe they are very clever and know what they are doing then either they think we are morons and won't join the dots OR they WANT us to know it's all a scam. I believe they do think we are morons (and let's face it, some deserve that label) and they are playing a game of poker face with a bad hand. It's a chance they are willing to take which shows they are desperate and time is running out. They want so bad for their gene technology to be the next big thing.

Here was a big clue last year that this was where they were going with it. [93]

---

[93] www.technologyreview.com/2021/02/05/1017366/messenger-rna-vaccines-covid-hiv/

THE BIG STORY: MRNA

The next act for messenger RNA could be bigger than covid vaccines

New messenger RNA vaccines to fight the coronavirus are based on a technology that could transform medicine. Next up: sickle cell and HIV.

By Antonio Regalado   February 5, 2021

The timing of this new release should also not be separated from the timely death of the original AIDS protagonist DR Luc Montaigne who challenged Gallo originally on his claim of HIV isolation. He also recently was very verbal about his theory that the covid shots would induce AIDS. His claims were a bit of the truth wrapped in innuendo.

What he was saying in essence was AIDS was iatrogenic.

There are SO many parallels to the AIDS 'pandemic' here that I find it hard to fathom having to point them out.

So they are twitching the curtains on the next act in this 'New World Hellth Order' and you need to be ready so you don't get sucked into another binge watch-worthy series of propaganda sales pitches. I covered what they can and, more importantly, can't do in 'The Amino Age' chapter.

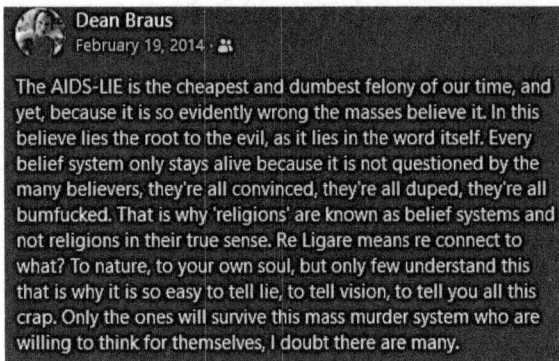

Dean Braus
February 19, 2014

The AIDS-LIE is the cheapest and dumbest felony of our time, and yet, because it is so evidently wrong the masses believe it. In this believe lies the root to the evil, as it lies in the word itself. Every belief system only stays alive because it is not questioned by the many believers, they're all convinced, they're all duped, they're all bumfucked. That is why 'religions' are known as belief systems and not religions in their true sense. Re Ligare means re connect to what? To nature, to your own soul, but only few understand this that is why it is so easy to tell lie, to tell vision, to tell you all this crap. Only the ones will survive this mass murder system who are willing to think for themselves, I doubt there are many.

Facebook post from 2014

Fake it till you make it is their usual game plan and they don't seem to care how many people they hurt as long as we keep buying the products and filling their coffers. I've been asked to write about AIDS but I haven't because it has all been done already. All we need to do is find the old evidence and re-release it like a broken down record or a Hollywood remake. I also briefly touched on the subject in the

'Contagion – Fact-Checked' chapter:

Another reason for re-introducing the HIV/AIDS story is to cover up the iatrogenic deaths which are about to skyrocket. This has been done over and over yet still their own data is pretty gob smacking. When you look at the 'official' figures you have to bear in mind these are only the figures they have to admit to. They cover up many iatrogenic deaths by blaming the 'disease' or 'virus', specifically in the case of cancer and heart disease, deaths from which are never blamed on the drugs. Even when it is blatantly obvious they are killing people it doesn't seem to tip the mainstream into pointing the finger. [94]

"If there is evidence that HIV causes AIDS, there should be scientific documents which either singly or collectively demonstrate that fact, at least with a high probability. There is no such document." – Dr. Kary Mullis, Biochemist, 1993 Nobel Prize for Chemistry.

"Up to today there is actually no single scientifically really convincing evidence for the existence of HIV. Not even once such a retrovirus has been isolated and purified by the methods of classical virology." – Dr. Heinz Ludwig Sanger, Emeritus Professor of Molecular Biology and Virology, Max-Planck-Institutes for Biochemistry, Munchen.

NOT A MYSTERY (DOCTORS ARE BAFFLED?)

Recently I've seen a growing number of 'news' reports claiming children are suffering from liver failure. The reports are scant on real information though. They do not mention ages, vaccine status, co-morbidities or anything. Nada. [95]

Newsweek

.S. | World | Business | Tech & Science | Culture | Autos | Sports | Health | Life | Opinion | Exper

NEWS

Hepatitis Outbreak Sees 17 Children Needing Liver Transplants, 1 Dying: WHO

BY FATMA KHALED ON 4/24/22 AT 4.35 PM EDT

---

[94] www.ourcivilisation.com/medicine/usamed/deaths.htm

[95] www.newsweek.com/hepatitis-outbreak-sees-17-children-needing-liver-transplants-1-dying-who-1700422

The few things they do mention though are mind numbing.

1. They claim the covid vaccine has been ruled out as a cause but zero information on how or why!!
2. They claim the culprit is another 'virus'.
3. They claim that the culprit is not the 'virus' alone there has to be a co-conspirator in the mix. Something else in combo with the 'virus' is triggering liver failure but no mention of what that might be.

OK when they start to spout utter nonsense my interest is piqued. If a virus is not the sole cause of a disease then it is not the cause of a disease. Just as they found Tuberculin in healthy people as well as sick people right at the start of the whole germ theory scam. This is why they invented the magical 'immune system' theory while it really should have just killed the germ theory outright.

The name of this 'virus' which may or may not be deadly (on its own) then?

Adenovirus.

Adeno stands for adenoids which is where they claim to have found this 'virus' back in the 50's.

So let's have a look at what they actually found: [96]

1. From the present evidence it appears that an unidentified, possibly new, tissue culture cytopathogenic agent has been isolated repeatedly from human adenoids undergoing spontaneous degeneration in tissue culture. The filter ability and the inability to cultivate the agent on bacteriological media and to demonstrate organisms in stained tissue culture preparations would indicate that the agent belongs to the group of viruses or rickettsial It is tentatively proposed to designate the agent as the "adenoid degeneration agent", abbreviated as "A.D. agent". 2. That the agent is derived from the adenoid tissue rather than from the nutrient media is indicated by the fact that some adenoids and all human embryonic tissues cultivated in the identical media and at the same time have not undergone degeneration, although they are susceptible to infection with the agent; also, repeated attempts to isolate the agents from adenoid cultures not demonstrating degeneration have been uniformly unsuccessful. 3. Further investigation is in progress to determine the relation of the agent to the adenoids and to study their possible role in human disease; particularly upper respiratory infections.

The very first line – "From the present evidence it appears that an unidentified, possibly new, tissue culture cytopathogenic agent has

---

[96] https://journals.sagepub.com/doi/abs/10.3181/00379727-84-20714

been isolated repeatedly from human adenoids undergoing spontaneous degeneration in tissue culture." So they put some mashed up adenoid tissue into a cell culture and the 'adenoid cells' started to degrade. Well taking cells out of their natural environment for one will cause that but they don't actually say whether they were from a living host or a dead one either. This is their proof that a virus is present!!! To this day the same pathetic proof is used over and over with no control or fulfilling of Koch's postulates.

Being as this went on in the early 50's shortly after the Enders paper sent all virology down the tissue culture path for 'isolating' and 'cultivating' supposed 'viruses' I think we can safely say it's another scam virus discovery just like the measles 'virus' discovery of Enders was proven to be in a court of law in 2017.

The 'agent', as they call it, comes FROM the adenoids so it is part of the human body and not an 'invading pathogen'. Why they classed it as a 'rickettsial' agent is anyone's guess. I thought at first that word was something to do with Rickets which is a malnutrition problem but no according to them it is something you get from a bite e.g. a tick bite. A parasite.

Now if we look on Wiki at what it has to say about this 'adenovirus' lots of interesting stuff pops out AND the page seems to have been edited JUST before this 'liver failure' story started hitting the newspapers.

Categories: Adenoviridae | Virus families

This page was last edited on 11 March 2022, at 22:52 (UTC).

According to the Wiki page this so-called 'virus' causes everything from strep throat to whooping cough and has been found in many animals including BATS (again) and even a mention of snakes (oh snake venom again) is in there but said to be 'poorly understood' (oh really?).

The infection section was to me the most interesting as they seem to have added every 'side effect' of the covid jabs in there as signs of 'adenovirus infection' – well what a coincidence!! [97]

"Most people recover from adenovirus infections by themselves, but people with immunodeficiency sometimes die of adenovirus infections, and – rarely – even previously healthy people can die of these infections. This may be because sometimes adenoviral infection can lead to cardiac disorders. For example, in one study, some cardiac samples of patients with dilated cardiomyopathy were positive for presence of adenovirus type 8.

Adenoviruses are often transmitted by expectoration (e.g. aerosols) but they can also be transmitted by contact with an infected person, or by virus particles left on objects such as towels and faucet handles. Some people with adenovirus gastroenteritis may shed the virus in their stools for months after getting over the symptoms. The virus can be passed through water in swimming pools that are not sufficiently chlorinated.

As with many other illnesses, good handwashing practice is one way to inhibit the person-to-person transmission of adenoviruses. Heat and bleach will kill adenovirus on objects."

Oh wait did I say everything? Funnily enough there is absolutely NO MENTION of it causing liver failure. Hmmm maybe they'll add that in tomorrow?

Oh and guess what, apparently there is no 'anti-viral' drug for adenovirus yet. (I didn't think those things were specific to certain viruses anyway?) Well let's see if they announce one in the next few weeks shall we, no doubt it's sitting waiting to be presented behind the curtains as we speak to add to the growing arsenal of useless but highly toxic drugs ending in 'vir'.

The next section of interest is this:

"Adenoviruses have long been a popular viral vector for gene therapy due to their ability to affect both replicating and non-replicating cells, accommodate large transgenes, and code for proteins without integrating into the host cell genome. More specifically, they are used as a vehicle to administer targeted therapy in the form of recombinant DNA or protein. This therapy has been found especially useful in treating monogenic disease (e.g cystic fibrosis, X-linked SCID, alpha1-antitrypsin deficiency) and cancer. In China, oncolytic adenovirus is an approved cancer treatment. Specific modifications on

---

[97] https://en.wikipedia.org/wiki/Adenoviridae

fiber proteins are used to target adenovirus to certain cell types, a major effort is made to limit hepatotoxicity and prevent multiple organ failure. Adenovirus dodecahedron can qualify as a potent delivery platform for foreign antigens to human myeloid dendritic cells (MDC), and that it is efficiently presented to MDC to M1-specific CD8+ T lymphocytes. Adenovirus has been used for delivery of CRISPR/Cas9 gene editing systems, but high immune reactivity to viral infection has posed challenges in use for patients."

So they've been using it in GENE THERAPY?!! It gets even better.

"Adenovirus have been used to produce viral vector Covid-19 vaccines. In four candidate Covid-19 vaccines…Ad5…serves as the 'vector' to transport the surface protein gene of SARS-Cov-2. The goal is to genetically express the spike glycoprotein of severe acute respiratory syndrome coronavirus 2."

So this adeno'virus', or whatever it really is, IS AN INGREDIENT in COVID vaccines (gene therapy) yet they are not telling us if these kids with liver failure have had the gene therapy shots?!

Lastly but not least one line that gives the game away here…

"Oncolytic adenovirus is an approved cancer treatment. Specific modifications on fiber proteins are used to target Adenovirus to certain cell types, **a major effort is made to limit hepatoxicity and prevent multiple organ failure**. Adenovirus dodecahedron can qualify as a potent delivery platform for foreign antigens to human myeloid dendritic cells." 'Hepatoxicity' means it is toxic to THE LIVER!! Hello!

Now do you see what they're up to? Now I want to see real data on whether these kids have had the covid shots or whether this is connected to the HepB shots they've started giving to newborns in the last few years which started the whole HIV malarkey in the 1980's. (The Wiki page even has mention of HIV and AIDS at the bottom just to add in the fear factor I'm sure.) It is one or the other of those two shots causing this and not some trumped up 'virus' again. The same old modus operandi over and over – invent new vaccine – create new disease – invent new vaccine – ad infinitum or until you wake the f up.

EVERYTHING YOU NEVER THOUGHT YOU'D NEED TO KNOW ABOUT MONKEYPOX

I actually can't believe I'm writing this. Debunking a potential plandemic of MONKEYPOX? How is this a thing? Yup the world has lost its marbles. It seems the majority of people do not look further than their TV screen for info, blindly believing every new fear-mongering campaign with actual relish, it has to be said.

Well as usual I will try to put this nonsense to bed, again. It is not hard to find the clues and the gaping holes in their narrative. They're not even bothering to hide the holes so I will show you where they are and what it means. Starting with the good ole CDC website:

> Monkeypox was first discovered in 1958 when two outbreaks of a pox-like disease occurred in colonies of monkeys kept for research, hence the name 'monkeypox.' The first human case of monkeypox was recorded in 1970 in the Democratic Republic of the Congo (DRC) during a period of intensified effort to eliminate smallpox. Since then, monkeypox has been reported in people in

Did you spot that? They 'discovered' monkeypox in humans during a VACCINATION campaign in Africa for SMALLPOX!! So for those who need it spelled out, they injected children with noxious substances supposedly to prevent smallpox so when some of them presented with 'smallpox' they had to deflect (as they always do) and invent a new diagnosis to cover up the vaccine damage.

Look at these pictures and tell me it's not 'smallpox'. [98]

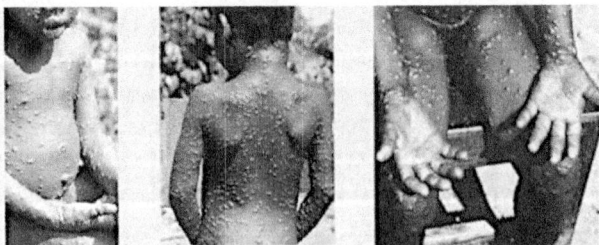

Another word for it is 'vaccinia'. It's hard to find accurate info on 'vaccinia' now as they have usurped the original meaning of the word to create yet another 'variant virus' from vaccine damage. Yes they've been doing that from the very first vaccine drive.

Original meaning of 'vaccinia' was:

Pathology

"An acute infection caused by inoculation with vaccina virus as a

---

[98] www.cdc.gov/poxvirus/monkeypox/index.html

prophylactic against smallpox, characterised by localized pustular eruptions."

Monkeypox was born out of vaccine damage just like Delta and Omicron were in 2021 and people keep falling for it. It's a never ending cycle. Next let's look at the origins (where did it come from) and holes in the official story on Wiki:

Monkeypox virus

"Monkeypox virus causes the disease in both humans and animals. **It was first identified by Preben von Magnus in 1958** as a pathogen of crab-eating macaque monkeys (Macaca fasicularis) being used as laboratory animals, **when two outbreaks of a smallpox-like disease occurred in colonies of monkeys kept for research.** The crab-eating macaque is often used for neurological experiments."

So originally it came from monkeys but wait, not wild monkeys happily monkeying around in the jungle. No, monkeys that had been ripped from their home and families, shipped in boxes for hundreds of miles and stuck in a medical laboratory. NOT a naturally occurring disease at all then.

Well what a surprise.

Let's have a look at the discoverer of monkeypox now and how he 'discovered' it – interesting stuff.

Preben von Magnus

"Preben Christian Alexander von Magnus (25 February 1912 – 09 August 1973) was a Danish virologist who is known for his research on influenza, polio vaccination and monkeypox. He gave his name to the **Von Magnus phenomenon**. In the 1950's, together with his wife, the virologist Herdis von Magnus, **he directed the first Danish vaccination programme against polio**. In 1958 he was **the first to confirm the identity of the monkeypox virus** and to describe monkeypox in laboratory crab-eating Macaques during two outbreaks of the disease in the summer and autumn of that year. In 1959 he was appointed director of Statens Serum Institut. He represented Denmark at the 1959 Pugwash Conferences on Science and World Affairs where **he explained that respiratory viruses such as influenza and the common cold were unsuitable as biological weapons."**

So basically we can derive from this that the man works in the vaccine industry so is well placed to orchestrate a cover-up of the damage done in Africa by their smallpox campaign so they could go on to commit even more atrocities there with the next vaccine.

I also highlighted the rather strange sentence about bio-weapons because it seemed out of place but might be relevant later. To me it looked like a possible 'fact-check' addition to gaslight the tinfoil hatters spouting the covid-biolab conspiracy. Turns out he said it at one of those elite type meetings they like to hold to make us think they're doing a great job running the world. Sort of like a G7 meeting but with a silly name. Pugwash hahaha. Apart from discovering monkeypox he seems to have discovered something else of interest. DIP's?

Von Magnus Phenomenon

"Despite the **inability to isolate them**, von Magnus **discovered defective interfering particles (DIP's) using the 'influenza virus system'**. He called them 'incomplete' or 'immature'. He found that when viruses were expanded at high doses, 'incomplete viruses' or 'particles' were produced and that these interfered with viral replication. This resulted in a reduction in the infectivity of influenza. The physiological interaction between DIP's and the host and the effect on the replication of infectious standard virus have since been studied."

So, in plain English, what he discovered was the more chemicals they added to the poor chick embryo's (that is what the 'influenza virus system' is, a fancy name for poisoning unborn chicks) the more cell debris was produced that didn't match up to a computer generated gene sequence he was trying to replicate. In other words the gene sequences didn't match what it said on the tin.

Just like they can invent a new disease to cover up their vaccine damage they can also invent new 'particles' when the particles don't do what they're supposed to do. No-one stops to think maybe the RNA isn't matching up because they've mixed it with other species and the 'viruses' don't replicate because there is no such thing!! They even admit it openly on the opening line – "inability to isolate them". So he isolated nothing. He made them up, just like they made up viruses.

A bit more of their concocted story to cover up the fact their virus theory is total bunkum:

Defective Interfering Particles (DIP's)

"Also known as defective interfering viruses, **DIP's are spontaneously generated virus mutants in which a critical portion of the particle's genome has been lost** due to defective replication or non-homologous recombination. The mechanism of their formation is presumed to be as a result of template-switching during replication of the viral genome, although non-replicative mechanisms involving direct ligation of genomic RNA fragments have also been proposed. DIP's are derived from and associated with their parent virus, and particles are classed as DIP's if they are rendered non-infectious due to at least one essential gene of the virus being lost or severely damaged as a result of the defection. A DIP can usually still penetrate host cells, but requires another fully functional virus particle (the 'helper' virus) to co-infect a cell with it, in order to provide the lost factors. DIP's were first observed as early as the 1950's by Von Magnus and Schlesinger, both working with influenza viruses. However, direct evidence for DIP's was only found in the 1960's by Hackett who noticed presence of 'stumpy' particles of vesicular stomatitis virus in electron micrographs and the formalization of DIP's terminology was in 1970 by Huang and Baltimore. **DIP's can occur within nearly every class of both DNA and RNA viruses both in clinical and laboratory settings, including poliovirus, SARS coronavirus, measles, alphaviruses, respiratory syncytial virus and influenza virus."**

This was all going on in the heyday of the newly emerging science of 'genetics' and this was one of the many hurdles they managed to crawl over backwards to explain away. None of the listed 'viruses' that this allegedly happens with have been isolated so the gene sequences they were working from were all 'dirty'. You'd think things would have changed by now in our high-tech world but no, it's still exactly the same as explained in this excellent article:

"Anyone claiming that the existence of a genome is proof of a purified/isolated 'virus' is completely mistaken. The contamination of genomes is admittedly a widespread problem and one that is only getting worse. While it is a well-known issue, contamination of the database has not been properly assessed nor corrected. The use of inaccurate and incomplete reference sequences has only further propagated the problem into a vicious perpetual cycle of erroneous genomes built upon erroneous genome." [99]

So it seems von Magnus is pretty good at plugging up holes in the narrative. Back to the monkeypox discovery on his page where the story differs slightly:

Monkeypox

"Naturally occurring pox infections in non-human primates were

---

[99] https://viroliegy.com/2022/01/24/genome-contamination-a-widespread-problem/

first reported by Rik Gispen in 1949. Due to the similar clinical appearances, some of these cases may have been due to monkeypox rather than smallpox.

In 1958, von Magnus was the first to confirm the identity of the monkeypox virus and to describe monkeypox in laboratory crab-eating Macaques during two outbreaks of the disease in the summer and autumn of that year. A little more than thirty cases of monkeys with monkeypox were reported **more than fifty days after their arrival by ship from Singapore**. There were no deaths and no monkey-to-human transmission. Not all the exposed monkeys exhibited the illness. **He isolated the virus from the monkey kidney tissue cell culture** and from the chorioallantoic membrane of chick embryos. The characteristic appearance of the virus led von Magnus to **elucidate** that it belonged to the smallpox-vaccinia group of Poxvirdae.

In 1968, the **WHO reported that it was not infrequent to observe outbreaks of suspected smallpox and monkeypox in laboratory monkeys at more than twenty-five biological institutions around the world** and that further research was warranted to assess susceptibility in humans.

It was not until 1970, more than ten years after von Magnus identified the virus, that monkeypox was first identified in humans."

Unlike the CDC which hinted at the monkeys not being in a lab but being 'held', here we see they were in fact in the lab thousands of miles away from home and for a month and a half already so plenty of time to start jabbing them with experimental vaccine concoctions then.

Again he didn't 'isolate' the monkey virus. He used the Enders method of poisoning cells in a petri dish and calling the damage a virus and the cell/mucus/blood soup an 'isolation'.

This method was thoroughly debunked by Stefan Lanka in the 2017 court case in Germany.

It is also noted that it was pretty common for the poor monkeys to display these horrible symptoms in vivisection labs all over the world. I'm sure the 'scientists were baffled' again huh?

Von Magnus also seems to be well connected in the vaccine production elite and making lots of money no doubt:

Danish polio vaccination programme

"Following **Jonas Salk's discovery of a polio** vaccine in the early 1950's, the United States sent details of polio vaccine manufacturing to those that requested it, with the permission of President Eisenhower. **Von Magnus and his wife Herdis were not only Salk's lifelong**

friends, but were also appointed by the Danish government to direct the vaccination of all 7 to 12 year olds. The Statens Serum Institut produced its own modified polio vaccine using techniques based on what the Von Magnus's had learnt in the spring of 1953, when they accepted an invitation to visit Salk's laboratory. Due to the limited supply of inactivated virus, the Danish institute administered the vaccine subcutaneously, requiring smaller doses."

In case you didn't already know, Salk's polio vaccine had to be discontinued because it CAUSED paralysis and death and von Magnus started injecting the vaccine to save money. Nice people then. Enough of him…let's go back to the monkeypox Wiki page to see how they got to marketing this 'new' disease:

"The virus was first discovered in monkeys (hence the name), **and in humans in 1970**. Almost 50 cases were reported between 1970 and 1979, with more than two thirds of these being from Zaire. The other cases originated from Liberia, Nigeria, Ivory Coast and Sierra Leone. **By 1986, over 400 cases in humans were reported**. Small viral outbreaks with a death rate in the range of 10% and a secondary human-to-human infection rate of about the same amount occur routinely in equatorial Central and West Africa. The primary route of infection is thought to be contact with the infected animals or their bodily fluids. The first reported outbreak outside of the African continent occurred in the United States in 2003 and in the Midwestern states of Illinois, Indiana and Wisconsin, with one occurrence in New Jersey."

Yeh they don't seem to be moving too fast on this one, maybe using the 'slowly, slowly catchy monkey' method huh? Only 400 'cases' in 16 years. Probably keeping it on the backburner for later, just in case.

This next bit is a doozy. They reckon that the smallpox vaccine will protect against monkeypox…

Prevention

"Vaccination against smallpox is **assumed to provide protection** against human monkeypox infection, **because they are closely related** viruses and the vaccine protects animals from experimental lethal monkeypox challenges. **This has not been conclusively demonstrated** in humans, because routine smallpox vaccination was discontinued following the eradication of smallpox."

Well sorry but doesn't that go against their whole germ theory of one germ for one disease? Why it normally takes 10 years to come up with a vaccine because it is so specific?? This makes no sense m'Lud.

It's bloody bonkers. Are they monkeying us around? Why not just give us one vaccine to rule them all if you can just use any old vaccine?

Wait a minute though, I know what they're playing at. This is the old problem-reaction-bad-solution game. Offer us the most dangerous vaccine ever produced (the first one yeh) so they can pull their brand new, shiny, waiting in the wings as we speak, new monkeypox vaccine. Ta-dah. Yes they have one already of course.

Now here comes another very recent little Wiki editing job. Monkeypox was not 'infectious' since the 1950's until suddenly now in 2022. Well ain't that something. Magic.

"The other genetic clade of MPVX occurs in Western Africa. The case fatality rate is less than 1%. **No human-to-human transmission was documented until the 2022 monkeypox outbreak in Europe**."

So now let's get to the absolute star of the show. The actual virus, where is it, what does it look like, how much does it weigh? Have they sorted out an artist to make the pretty CGI pic everyone loves?

Read the paper claiming the 'isolation' of the monkeypox virus in 1972 here. (Told ya von Magnus didn't do it). [100]

Firstly antibodies are NO indication of ANY virus as they are not specific, even if they were there is no test to tell them apart and frankly no proof they do anything they say they do. (See 'Anti-Bodies Again' chapter for more on that).

As you can see from the last line they 'distinguished' a virus that was different from smallpox by looking at poisoned unborn pig kidney cells. No classification/isolation/control group and certainly no Koch's postulates fulfilled. Very shoddy work. Nothing to see here, move along.

THERE IS NO MONKEYPOX VIRUS! But let's sell it anyway...

Monkeypox even had its very own 'Event 201'. [101]

Just like at Event 201 they lay out what they expect to happen (or is it what they would LIKE to happen?) and they pretty much followed the script for covid so maybe we should have a look at what exactly they WANT to happen.

Aha, now I see where the bio-weapon link comes in that Mr von

---

[100] https://pubmed.ncbi.nlm.nih.gov/4340219/

[101] www.nti.org/wp-content/uploads/2021/11/NTI_Paper_BIO-TTX_Final.pdf (Page 10 is where the plot is – spoiler alert).

Magnus was harping on about at his Pugwash meeting. They are gonna go with the old bio-weapon made in a lab ruse that all the controlled opposition were screaming about last time. So now they are being promoted from tin-foil hat conspiracy nuts to working for the dark side. Nice bit of mental priming they did there.

For this to work for them the whole world needs to be bat-shit crazy/hypnotized or they will push through the WHO Pandemic Treaty and then it won't matter if no-one believes them, they will have the power to do it anyway. It's not too late to stop them. Or is it?

First Childhood Death From Mystery Hepatitis In Ireland

When I first reported on this story there was scant information and now they have ramped it up with their much beloved reporting of a death. Death creates fear like nothing else. I know because I felt it too back in the 80's when they were doing a meningitis scare to sell their new meningitis jab. That was probably the closest I came to caving.

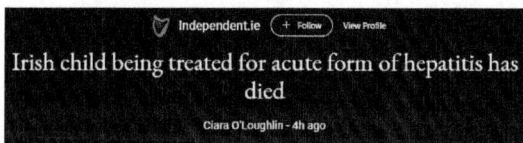

Independent.ie (+ Follow)   View Profile

Irish child being treated for acute form of hepatitis has died

Ciara O'Loughlin - 4h ago

Reading through this news piece there are a few clues. Firstly:

Over the past 10 weeks, six probable cases of children with hepatitis of unknown cause have been detected in Ireland.

Now what happened about 10 weeks previously? Pretty obvious to me but for those who might not have put 2+2 together, look at the news article on the BBC website dated 3rd January 2022 'covid jab offered to five to 11-year old children in Ireland'. [102]

In the last article before this death there was no mention of covid jabs at all which is suspicious wouldn't you say? As is always the case they will look at ANYTHING BUT their own drugs as a cause of sickness. How can they legitimately take that stance when it is officially, by their own admission, the leading cause of death today? Iatrogenesis. Look it up, it means 'death by doctor'.

---

[102] www.bbc.com/news/world-europe-59857507

This time though they DO mention the convid jabs. Maybe because people WERE putting 2+2 together and they needed to squash that thinking.

> The public health expert said medics could rule out any link between the cases and vaccinations for Covid-19 with "absolute certainty", as in most cases in the UK the children had not received the vaccine.

Most people reading that would be satisfied, but not me. Firstly they are using word from the UK to rule out the jabs being the cause in IRELAND?? Not very scientific!!

Oh it can't be the jabs coz Dr Knowitall from England told me so in the brown envelope I received last night? Hmm.

Secondly the UK Knowitall stated that "in MOST cases the children had not received the vaccine." OK so if we take that as true (and I suspect it is not true) 'most' means more than half, like 51% so almost half COULD have been vaccinated and even then, if you remember, they were calling people with only one jab as opposed to two, unvaccinated during the adult vaccine drive. So I'd take that statement with two dollops of salt myself.

Yet again though they are not giving us the age of the child, what 'treatments' they were given or the specific dead child's vaccine status. HIGHLY SUSPICIOUS!!

So what is the general protocol treatment for acute hepatitis? Funny you should ask because it happens to be those lovely 'anti-viral' drugs again. These are the new cash cows for the pharma companies as the old 'antibiotics' are A. not working so well and B. patents must be running out by now so no longer raking in the big bucks.

So if the jab doesn't do enough damage to the liver the treatments certainly will.

"Hepatitis B Treatment & Management: Medscape Reference
Any patient with acute HBV disease needs to be treated with first-line oral therapy, such as tenofovir disoproxil fumarate (TDF) or entecavir (ETV). Patients with acute hepatitis should be monitored with blood tests in order to document biochemical improvement (see Workup)." [103]

This time though we DO get a taste of the agenda behind this 'mystery illness' and its reporting around the world.

It is to boost the sales of the CHILDHOOD COVID SHOTS!

Obviously parents were being too hesitant this time, and rightly so.

---

[103] emedicine.medscape.com/article/177632-treatment

This line appeared on one article (Microsoft news) but not the other (Irish Times):

"If you have children that haven't been vaccinated at all and haven't had covid its worth considering maybe it's a good idea to get them vaccinated if you haven't done up to this point."

So there you have it. Give us one dead child and we will boost your sales to the moon to now terrified parents!!

Meanwhile the 'experts' will continue hunting around for a bogus scapegoat cause down at the biolabs where I'm sure they've got some artist working on a pretty picture of a 'novel' rhinovirus. Just remember they've always told us rhino-viruses (word means 'nose virus') were the cause of the common cold. You just can't make this shit up I tell you.

One other thing worth noting here is the HepB jab which has been snuck into one of the multi-jabs given to children in Ireland (and UK) in the last few years. I have always been of the opinion that the two big cases in 2018 of two specific children dying (Charlie Gard 2017 & Alfie Evans 2018) were the results of a trial of the HepB shots in the UK.

They eventually claimed their deaths were due to a DNA disease which is a bit like the old doctors diagnosis of 'a virus' but with even less proof. In other words utter bullshit but hey, at least it wasn't the vaccines huh??!! Notice the throwaway line that the jab is 'also' for babies of 'infected' mothers etc.? Yes, because that was all it was originally meant to be for. What infection? HIV!!

And so we come full circle to the drive to get everyone HIV tested again. Dizzy yet? Are you joining the dots yet?

There are NO VIRUSES attacking the liver. The liver's function is to remove toxins from the body. The most common cause of liver failure is an overload of toxins or poisons, the most obvious being alcohol. We all know this so how is it that they can't see what is causing it in non-alcoholics? It's pretty obvious to me. DRUGS including vaccines.

"The liver's main job is to filter the blood coming from the digestive tract, before passing it to the rest of the body. The liver also detoxifies chemicals and metabolizes drugs. As it does so, the liver secretes bile that ends up back in the intestines. The liver also makes proteins important for blood clotting and other functions." Snippet from WebMD [104]

---

[104] www.webmd.com/digestive-disorders/picture-of-the-liver

This quote from an N.D. says it all for me.

"When liver toxicity develops, then as long as sufficient vitality exists, the body will attempt remedial action in the form of liver inflammation, a condition that medical authorities refer to as Hepatitis. ('Hep' meaning liver, and 'itis' meaning inflammation). The purpose of inflammation is to reduce the liver's toxicity level and to carry out healing and repair. What I am therefore saying is that Hepatitis is not the disease, but in fact, the cure." – Ian Sinclair, N.D.

Anti-Bodies Again

1. Antibodies are very important for our immune system in getting over viral and bacterial diseases. We make non-specific IgM Antibodies (Ab) initially then specific IgG Ab later. Once we make IgG we are immune for life against that pathogen.

2. An example of this is with mumps, mumps is caused by a virus, we get the disease once, make IgG antibodies and are immune for life.

3. Another example is measles, we test for IgG and prove we are immune for life, well except that in a Supreme Court case in Germany it was shown that the measles virus doesn't exist, never mind.

4. Another example is chickenpox, we get chicken pox once and never again due to IgG antibodies, except if we get shingles which is also chickenpox, but well that's different.

5. If we have AIDS we test for the presence of Ab, if we have them we know for sure that we have a deadly virus which will soon kill us. That's because the HI virus is 'smart' and knows how to evade the Ab unlike the mumps virus which is stupid and doesn't. The measles virus doesn't exist and the chickenpox virus is smart-ish.

6. Another example is Hep C, again if your liver is falling apart you can be tested for Ab and if they are positive it means you have a deadly virus which is eating your liver. This is clearly another example of a smart virus.

7. With rhino virus, the cause of the common cold, we, naturally develop antibodies to the virus, but this virus is very smart (seeing as how it jumped to humans as a result of the unfortunate tendency of Africans to eat rhinos) and many of us get colds year after year in spite of the presence of antibodies.

8. Similarly the influenza virus is very, very smart and unlike the measles virus which not only doesn't exist but has remained constant in its non-existence for centuries, the flu virus changes its form yearly. This is undoubtedly because the flu virus is so smart it has included flu vaccine companies in its stock market portfolio. I wish I were as smart as the flu virus.

9. If you have symptoms of Lyme's disease and you test for the presence of Ab and show them to your infectious disease

doctor and tell him you tested positive for antibodies which means you have Lyme disease, he will throw you out of the office and call you a fucking lunatic. That's because the presence of Ab don't mean anything in Lyme's disease

10. If you have covid and you test positive for Ab it means you either had the virus or you didn't have the virus. Also, it is clear evidence that you were either sick or not sick. That's because the corona virus is so smart that it can trick you into either making Ab or not to throw off the immunologists.

Hope this makes it perfectly clear – Tom Cowan, M.D.

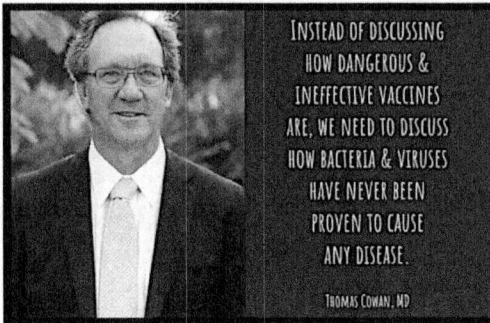

INSTEAD OF DISCUSSING HOW DANGEROUS & INEFFECTIVE VACCINES ARE, WE NEED TO DISCUSS HOW BACTERIA & VIRUSES HAVE NEVER BEEN PROVEN TO CAUSE ANY DISEASE.

THOMAS COWAN, MD

If you've read this far hold onto your hat for some serious stuff...

From The Independent: "Covid patients in the UK are to be treated with man-made antibodies that prevent and fight coronavirus infection after approval was granted by the medicines regulator. Health secretary Sajid Javid said the treatment, which was used on former US president Donald Trump after he fell with Covid-19, would be rolled out through the NHS "as soon as possible".

'Antibodies', hmm really...artificial ones at that. NOT good.

"The Medicines and Healthcare products Regulatory Agency (MHRA) said the clinical trial data they had assessed has shown Ronapreve may be used to prevent infection, treat symptoms of acute Covid-19 infection and can reduce the likelihood of being admitted to hospital due to the virus." [105]

Addendum 30/01/2022

The monoclonal-antibody treatment has hit a dead end (literally). Despite protests from the likes of Natural News and Tucker Carlson

---

[105] www.independent.co.uk/news/health/covid-antibody-treatment-uk-nhs-b1905837.html

the utter madness of this experimental 'treatment' has had to be stopped.

WTF is a 'passive vaccine'? Is it a bit like a 'live virus' I wonder? [106]

But what ARE antibodies really? Do they even exist or do what they say they do? No they don't.

We all know that the whole science of vaccines is built on antibody production. That is how they measure their effectiveness too.

So if they are wrong about antibodies then they are wrong about immunity and vaccines have no place in medicine.

They ARE wrong about antibodies…

ANTIBODIES DEBUNKED

A collection of quotes from doctors and scientists on what they think antibodies are and what they are not:

The whole vaccine business is built on the very dodgy foundation of a theory called 'the immune system'. Vaccines are tested for efficacy by measuring antibody levels which everyone believes equates to some form of 'immunity' to reinfection. But what if antibodies were not what we've been told?

Adam Finn, a pediatric expert at Sheffield Children's Hospital said: "the normal trials on a new vaccine were not possible in Britain because of the relatively small numbers of people who contracted the disease. Instead scientists had tested whether the vaccine produced sufficient antibodies" **– Media report on meningitis C vaccine**. [107]

"From repeated medical investigations, it would seem that antibodies are about as useful as a black eye in protecting the victim from further attacks. The word 'antibody' covers a number of even less intelligible words, quaint relics of Erlich's side-chain theory, which the greatest of experts, McDonagh, tells us is 'essentially unintelligible.'

Now that the old history, mythology and statistics of vaccination have been exploded by experience, the business has to depend more upon verbal dust thrown in the face of the lay public. The mere layman,

---

[106] www.unite4truth.com/post/real-reason-monoclonal-antibodies-lost-fda-eua-associate-drug-fail-safety-trial-lethal-side-effect

[107] http://whale.to/v/meningitis5.html

assailed by antibodies, receptors, haptophores, etc., is only too pleased to give up the fight and leave everything to the experts. This is just what they want, especially when he is so pleased that he also leaves them lots and lots of real money. The whole subject of immunity and antibodies is, however, so extremely complex and difficult, especially to the real experts, that it is a relief to be told that the gaps in their knowledge of such things are still enormous. We can obtain some idea of the complexity of the subject from The Integrity of the Human Body, by Sir Macfarlane Burnet. He calls attention to the fact – the mystery – that some children can never develop any antibodies at all, but can nevertheless go through a typical attack of, say, measles, make a normal recovery and show the normal continuing resistance to reinfection.

Furthermore, we have heard for years past of attempts made to relate the amount of antibody in patients to their degree of immunity to infection. The results have often been so farcically chaotic, so entirely unlike what was expected, that the scandal has had to be hushed up – or put into a report, which is much the same thing (vide M.R.C. Report, No. 272, May 1950, A Study of Diphtheria in Two Areas of Great Britain, now out of print). The worst scandal, however, is that the radio is still telling the schools that the purpose of vaccinating is to produce antibodies. The purpose of vaccinating is to make money!" **– Lionel Dole.** [108]

"Human trials generally correlate "antibody" responses with protection – that is if the body produces antibodies (proteins) which bind to vaccine components, then it must be working and safe. Yet Dr. March says antibody response is generally a poor measure of protection and no indicator at all of safety. "Particularly for viral diseases, the 'cellular' immune response is all important, and antibody levels and protection are totally unconnected." **– Private Eye 24/1/2002.** [109]

A 'titre' is a measurement of how much antibody to a certain virus (or other antigen) is circulating in the blood at that moment. Titres are usually expressed in a ratio, which is how many times they could dilute the blood until they couldn't find antibodies anymore. So let's say they could dilute it two times only and then they didn't find anymore, that would be a titre of 1:2. If they could dilute it a thousand times before they couldn't find any antibody, then that would be a titre of 1:1000.

[108] http://whale.to/v/dole.html
[109] http://whale.to/v/mmr445.html

A titre test does not and cannot measure immunity, because immunity to specific viruses is reliant not on antibodies, but on memory cells, which we have no way to measure. Memory cells are what prompt the immune system to create antibodies and dispatch them to an infection caused by the virus it 'remembers.' Memory cells don't need 'reminders' in the form of re-vaccination to keep producing antibodies. (Science, 1999; "Immune system's memory does not need reminders"). **– ACCESS to JUSTICE. MMR10 – IN EUROPE**. [110]

"The theory that the creation of antibodies in the blood indicates that protection against disease has been established is not supported by experience. The Medical Research Council's Report on Diphtheria Outbreaks in Gateshead and Dundee, published in 1950, showed that many of the persons actually in hospital with diphtheria had far more anti-toxin in their blood than was said to be required for complete protection against diphtheria, whilst nurses and others in close contact with diphtheria infection and without sufficient anti-toxin remained immune." [111] **– The Brains Of The Inoculated - from a 1957 speech by Lily Loat, Secretary of the National Anti-Vaccination League**.

In order to better grasp the issue of vaccine effectiveness, it would prove helpful for us to go back to the early theoretical foundation upon which current vaccination and disease theories originated. In simplest terms, the theory of artificial immunization postulates that by giving a person a mild form of a disease, via the use of specific foreign proteins, attenuated viruses, etc., the body will react by producing a lasting protective response e.g., antibodies, to protect the body if or when the real disease comes along. This primal theory of disease prevention originated by Paul Ehrlich – from the time of its inception – has been subject to increasing abandonment by scientists of no small stature. For example not long after the Ehrlich theory came into vogue, W.H. Manwaring, then Professor of Bacteriology and Experimental Pathology at Leland Stanford University observed: "I believe that there is hardly an element of truth in a single one of the basic hypothesis embodied in this theory. My conviction that there was something radically wrong with it arose from a consideration of the almost universal failure of therapeutic methods based on it. Twelve years of

---

[110] http://whale.to/vaccines/access_to_justice.html
[111] http://whale.to/vaccines/loat1.html

study with immuno-physical tests have yielded a mass of experimental evidence contrary to, and irreconcilable with the Ehrlich theory, and have convinced me that his conception of the origin, nature, and physiological role of the specific 'antibodies' is erroneous.

To afford us with a continuing historical perspective of events since Manwaring's time, we can next turn to the classic work on auto-immunity and disease by Sir MacFarlane Burnett, which indicates that since the middle of this century the place of antibodies at the center stage of immunity to disease has undergone "a striking demotion." For example, it had become well known that children with agammaglobulinemia – who consequently have no capacity to produce antibody – after contracting measles, (or other zymotic diseases) nonetheless recover with long-lasting immunity. In his view it was clear "that a variety of other immunological mechanisms are functioning effectively without benefit of actively produced antibody."

The kind of research which led to this a broader perspective on the body's immunological mechanisms included a mid-century British investigation on the relationship of the incidence of diphtheria to the presence of antibodies. The study concluded that there was no observable correlation between the antibody count and the incidence of the disease." "The researchers found people who were highly resistant with extremely low antibody count, and people who developed the disease who had high antibody counts. (According to Don de Savingy of IDRC, the significance of the role of multiple immunological factors and mechanisms has gained wide recognition in scientific thinking. (For example, it is now generally held that vaccines operate by stimulating non-humeral mechanisms, with antibody serving only as an indicator that a vaccine was given, or that a person was exposed to a particular infectious agent.)

In the early 1970's we find an article in the Australian Journal of Medical Technology by medical virologist B. Allen (of the Australian Laboratory of Microbiology and Pathology, Brisbane) which reported that although a group of recruits were immunized for Rubella, and uniformly demonstrated antibodies, 80 percent of the recruits contracted the disease when later exposed to it.

Similar results were demonstrated in a consecutive study conducted at an institution for the mentally disabled. Allen, in commenting on herb research at a University of Melbourne seminar, stated that "one must wonder whether the decision to rely on herd immunity might not have to be re-thought."

As we proceed to the early 1980's, we find that upon investigating unexpected and unexplainable outbreaks of acute infection among 'immunized' persons, mainstream scientists have begun to seriously question whether their understanding of what constitutes reliable immunity is in fact valid. For example, a team of scientist writing in the New England Journal of Medicine provide evidence for the position that immunity to disease is a broader bio-ecological question then the factors of artificial immunization or serology. They summarily concluded: "It is important to stress that immunity (or its absence) cannot be determined reliable on the basis of history of the disease, history of immunization, or even history of prior serologic determination."

Despite these significant shifts in scientific thinking, there has unfortunately been little actual progress made in terms of undertaking systematically broad research on the multiple factors which undergird human immunity to disease, and in turn building a system of prevention that is squarely based upon such findings.

It seems ironic that as late as 1988 James must still raise the following basic questions. "Why doesn't medical research focus on what factors in our environment and in our lives weaken the immune system? Is this too simple? too ordinary? too undramatic? Or does it threaten too many vested interests ?" – **Dr. Obomsawin M.D**. [112]

Antibodies are proteins (produced by the 'immune system'.)

"Antibodies are, in reality, soluble blood proteins, which play a central role in the healing of wounds. In a test tube containing an appropriate concentration of acids and bases, minerals and solvents, these blood proteins, also called globulins, will bind arbitrarily from other proteins. Thus you can make any sample taken from an animal or a person test arbitrarily positive or negative." – **Lanka interview 2005**

(So if they are there to heal wounds it makes sense they would be around poisoned, dying cells, right? The theory that they are specific to every disease has been disproven, there are only a few different proteins they call 'anti-bodies' whereas there are infinite types of 'viruses' by their own admission.)

Definition from the Online Etymology Dictionary:

---

[112] https://web.archive.org/web/20001215233300/http://www.whal e.to/vaccines/obomsawin.html

Antibody (n.) "substance developed in blood as an antitoxin" 1901, a hybrid formed from **anti** "against" + **body**. Probably a translation of German Antikörper, condensed from a phrase such as anti-toxischer Körper "anti-toxic body" (1891).

This may be news to many but it is in fact long known in medical circles which means the vaccine industry is committing fraud (apart from murder) and we really need a moratorium on the whole 'vaccine' issue NOW.

Antibodies – A Closer Look

(I wrote this after my own translation of an article by Stefan Lanka called 'The Misinterpretation of Antibodies') [113]

It's important to understand what antibodies are because the vaccine industry use them as their indication that vaccines work. They claim that measuring the amount of antibodies in the blood (a titre) is an indication of 'immunity' after a vaccine (except in the case of HIV lol, we'll get to that later.)

The sudden increase in titre though is really an indicator that the body has been poisoned. Antibodies are a kind of protein (globulin) which repairs damage to cells and causes blood to clot.

They claim that antibodies are specific. That is also not true, all the talk of binding and receptors is nonsense, globulins will bind to anything depending on the level of acid in the tissues/blood.

How do we know this? Because they can manipulate what they bind to by manipulating the acid levels with detergents.

For example, pregnancy causes a massive uptick in globulins which is why they say pregnancy can produce an HIV positive diagnosis (but so can flu and other things). The reason a pregnant woman has lots of globulins is to keep the placenta constantly sealed as it grows.

All vaccines are approved for efficacy based on this counting of antibodies/globulins which they call 'seroconversion' after the vaccine. The whole industry hangs on this massive lie that antibodies = immunity. This information is out there in the open and well known in medicine. In April 2001 'Telegram of Medicines' stated "Vaccine-induced titre increases are also unreliable substitutes for efficacy."

The RKI (Robert Koch Institute) wrote: "For some vaccine-

---

[113] https://northerntracey213875959.wordpress.com/2020/11/26/the-misinterpretation-of-antibodies/

preventable diseases (e.g. pertussis) there is no reliable serological correlate that could be used as a surrogate marker for existing immunity. Furthermore, the antibody concentration does not allow conclusions to be drawn about any kind of cellular immunity."

Prof. Heininger, a long-standing member of STIKO (permanent vaccination commission) wrote: "It is neither necessary nor useful to determine efficacy by blood sampling and antibody determination after a vaccination has been carried out. An antibody determination does not provide a reliable indication of the presence or absence of vaccination protection, and it is too expensive."

An example of becoming sick despite vaccination: A 14-year-old boy who had received immunisation in childhood and a booster against tetanus six months earlier when he developed tetanus. Laboratory tests revealed antibodies so high that, according to their standards he should have been protected. But he was not! This shows their theory that antibodies are 'protective magic bullets' is wrong. When this became obvious the RKI coined the new term 'non-protective' antibodies.

Not to halt the gravy train but to instead boost sales they also invented 'booster shots' on the back of this finding. Example using the MMR: "There are not only false-negative IgG antibody results but unfortunately also false-positive results. This must be put to parents so that they understand that a positive laboratory result does not certify protection and that they are much better advised to give their child a second dose of MMR." – Prof. Heininger of STIKO (2016)

If no one can say exactly what titre level indicates protection, why is the approval of a vaccine based on this test? To put it simply, the connection between antibodies and immunity is a myth.

Another example of their bumbling on titre levels – they claim that in the cases of HiB and measles much lower antibody levels will protect against catching the disease, (protection from disease) than the level to prevent transmission to others (protection from infection). As there is still no scientific proof of a measles virus, the question arises as to how antibodies can protect from measles when that pathogen has not yet been proven to exist. They have put the horse before the cart here. By measuring some 'antibodies' they're indirectly claiming to have a pathogen. Magic!

High antibody titres after a vaccine only occurs because of the 'adjuvants'. Many people wonder why they have to put adjuvants in vaccines at all – well the secret is, no adjuvant = no antibody count. What does that tell us? What is an adjuvant you ask? Usually some kind of protein or heavy metal.

People with herpes develop antibodies, which they say are 'specific', yet herpes can flare up time and time again. Where is the immunity? Then there is the curious case of HIV. How is it possible that their story about antibodies was turned on its head into high antibody levels being deemed a bad thing in this one case – HIV?

'Circulating antibodies alone do not provide reliable protection' this has been orthodox medical knowledge for many decades. On the other hand, the proof of efficacy in the approval of vaccines is based solely on the proof of the allegedly protective (sometimes?) antibody count/titres.

If antibodies are found after vaccination, conventional medicine tells us that the patient is now protected. However they don't tell us that people can be ill despite high antibody counts and people without antibodies can be perfectly healthy. When HIV antibodies are detected a diagnosis of fatally ill, or at least will become fatally ill, is the new normal.

The name anti-body is a contradiction in terms. The 'bodies' called immunoglobulins do exist. Among other things they play a role in the coagulation and cross-linking of proteins. The word 'anti' assumes that the immunoglobulins can only bind to certain proteins – all experiments ever performed however, rule this out. Whether or not binding takes place depends on the environment/terrain and state of the proteins: Whether acidic or basic, i.e. oxidised or reduced. Every scientist who has carried out such experiments or studied them knows this.

How do they test for antibodies?

First, the blood is separated from its cells and the larger proteins by centrifuge. It's the blood serum that is tested. The lab technician is then told what he/she is supposed to find in the serum (e.g. antibodies to 'HIV'). Then the sleight of hand comes. They have to add the corresponding, pharmaceutically produced, patented substance whose ingredients are kept secret by the government and the Paul-Ehrlich-Institute. The lab technician is told that the test kit contains one or more proteins which correspond to the shape of the microbe they are seeking. Under these lab conditions the shape of the proteins could not correspond to that of any claimed microbe, because the proteins are no longer in their natural environment. This is called denaturation of the proteins. These secret proteins are named 'antigens' which can detect the antibodies. Magic again!

The test kit also contains dyes and substances that will produce a 'positive' result. The apparatus, into which the whole thing is then placed, is calibrated again with substances whose composition is kept secret and which are monitored by the aforementioned Paul Ehrlich Institute.

If there is a measurable reaction the test is positive.

Once they have their antibody count/titre then they seem to become confused as there is no scientific standard for titres and the measurements are never comparable. In other words there are no scientific criteria whatsoever as to when a titre can, should, may or might be called 'immune protection'.

The fact that there are about 5% of people whose blood, under laboratory conditions, show little or no immunoglobulins, is never discussed or investigated.

These people are called 'non-responsive' to vaccination and are poisoned with more and more boosters following their delusional compulsion. Blood group AB was invented for these 5% of non-responders. Did you know blood groups were all based on antibody tests?

The contradiction that arose for the dogma of blood groups was first dismissed by the discovery of a rhesus factor and resulted in a continuous introduction of thousands of new sub-blood groups.

Feli Popescu wrote an interesting article – 'Rhesus factor, blood groups, blood plasma, anti-D prophylaxis'. This article shows extreme inconsistencies and discrepancies in how science works. You can also see in the article how the antibody theory is debunked. I can't include it in this book but you can find it online. [114]

A few awkward facts:

- Alternating 'foreign' intestinal bacteria exist side by side with 'immune cells' which are supposed to launch a specific defence against them. If there were specific antibodies, the intestinal flora should never be able to change. But it does.

- Humans, mammals, bony fish and sharks exist. They all produce immunoglobulins. If they were specific antibodies, their offspring would be destroyed and breast

---

[114] www.northerntracey213875959.wordpress.com/2020/12/27/rhes us-factoranalysis-of-rhesus-factor-claims-author-feli-popescuin/

milk would be toxic.

- During development of humans and animals or in shock and in old age, new proteins are produced. Since, according to the immune hypothesis, 'foreign' and 'own' proteins are recognized by the thymus in earliest childhood and 'antibodies' are sorted from 'own' proteins, proteins which occur later, such as hormones in puberty etc., would automatically lead to allergy, autoimmune diseases, destruction and death. This is however not the case either.

- Anti-bodies against viruses which do not exist at all cannot exist in principle either. An antibody can only be claimed if the body has been detected. It is claimed that many viral antibodies can be detected (by magic tests) without the virus being able to be verified scientifically.

- Antibodies are formed in 'infectious diseases' and the detection of antibodies is proof of protection against the disease. According to orthodox medicine, HIV-positivity (antibodies) should be the best protection against AIDS however they claim the opposite in this one case.

Every test measures what the test measures, only nobody knows exactly what the test measures. The tests react non-specifically to proteins. No test can detect anti-'bodies' if the underlying 'body' has never been detected.

ANTIBODIES – Reality versus belief.

THE VACCINATION BELIEF – Vaccination = Antibody = Protection = Long life and health.

THE REALITY – Small proteins are called globulins. These globulins are produced by the body when cells need to be multiplied, repaired or newly formed.

The whole vaccination business is based on globulins' ability to bind with other proteins and molecules.

Did you know so-called 'antibodies' were once called 'healing bodies' by Emil von Behring 1892 and 'magic balls' by Paul Ehrlich who also coined the term 'magic bullet'.

The powerful aluminium adjuvant from Gardasil came under question during a case in 2019 – during the trial it was stated: "Among vaccinologists, it's axiomatic that the duration of immunity correlates directly to the toxicity of the adjuvant; **the more toxic the adjuvant,**

the longer the duration of immunity." [115]

That's perfectly put. The toxins are supposed to boost the antibody levels so that something can be measured and which a vaccine cannot produce without these adjuvants.

The deception starts where the measured value is pretended to be immunity, because in reality it only indicates the degree of poisoning, not the effectiveness of a vaccine according to their key-lock theory and the fairy tales of viral load, antigens etc.

Correspondence between Hans Tolzin and Robert Koch Institute (RKI) on the topic of antibodies:

This correspondence shows that the RKI does not consider the antibody level (titre) the sole criterion for protection.

RKI writes on 01.02.2005 "Neither the RKI nor the STIKO consider the level of antibody concentration the sole criterion for immunity and do not define it as such. Cellular immunity (immunological memory), which is particularly important for long-term immunity, is not dependent on the detectable antibody titres and therefore antibody titres only serve as 'surrogate markers' for immunity"… However, undetectable or low antibody titres are not proof of non- immunity."

So we see, no matter if antibodies are measured or not, according to the RKI there is protection from non-existent as well as existing antibodies. Since we know that these 'antibodies' are created when cells are poisoned/ destroyed, it can't be stated that a virus is the cause, but rather poisoning by a vaccination and your harmful adjuvants.

Hans Tolzin asks: "If, as you say, the level of antibody concentration does not show a reliable clue to immunity, how can it be the sole criterion for proof of benefit in vaccine approval? I don't understand."

Reply from RKI: "Dear Mr. Tolzin, we have replied at length. For capacity reasons we cannot continue the discussion. Yours sincerely"

Even the best liars lose the plot when confronted with the truth.

With HIV, the complete nonsense of antibodies was finally revealed.

Der Spiegel wrote: "In HIV-infected persons scientists were able to detect above-average numbers of antibodies against various viruses. This could be explained by the fact that the HI virus can weaken the immune system and make the affected persons more susceptible to

[115] https://childrenshealthdefense.org/news/court-hears-gardasil-science-and-moves-forward/

further infections."

HIV, therefore tells us antibodies are more likely to indicate that a person is weakened, even though he or she has extremely high antibody levels. In principle, he should be a highly protected person. The basic thesis was not even questioned, although in the case of HIV the dissenting voices were extremely loud.

The conclusion:

The state authorities are not aware of any scientific evidence that antibodies protect from illness so they invoke a spell to blind you with science-waffle. The employees of the authorities assume their masters know what they are talking about and adopt a blind faith attitude which trickles down to all us minions at the bottom.

Rules on how to keep the gravy train rolling:

Use surrogates like antibodies to claim protection, with no scientific basis nor confirmation of the claim.

Use a DNA 'test' (PCR) which cannot provide proof of any virus but is a manipulation tool that has never been validated.

Use leading consultants who have already been convicted of fraud.

What did Horst Seehofer say to ZDF (like the German BBC) about the power of the pharmaceutical lobby?

"The pharmaceutical lobby is too strong, this has been the case for 30 years, it is not possible to introduce meaningful changes because these structures are so powerful that the politicians cannot influence them". Seehofer says: *"I can only tell you that this is the case and it is working very effectively"*

Reporter's question: "How is it possible that the pharmaceutical lobby is stronger than the politicians of a country?

Seehofer: *"I can't disagree with you there…"*

The term 'immunity' should be replaced by a term like 'healing power'. Healing ability cannot be produced by any kind of vaccination, it is an ability of the whole being (body-mind-spirit) and depends on many factors.

Anaphylaxis

The Real Bio-Weapon

In 2020 I revisited some old research I'd uncovered during my early vaccine research days. I'd been searching for the cause of the sudden growth in allergies, in particular the infamous peanut allergy.

I got some info from a nurse I knew on Care2 who sent me an obscure paper which listed peanut oil as one of the ingredients in one of the childhood schedule vaccines. This was the proof I'd been searching for and which confirmed my suspicions that vaccines WERE the cause of allergies. More recently articles have appeared documenting the allergy-vaccine connection like this one on Vaccinetruth.org. [116]

This was at a time when information was much harder to come by and to my knowledge no-one else was joining the dots between vaccines and allergies. Yet the proof was already out there and had been known in the realms of science for 100 years at least from the Nobel prize winning work of Charles Richet. I did not uncover this until years later, well before I started putting my thoughts down in articles. Charles Richet's work has been well hidden for a long time. Ask your doctor if they've heard of him. I doubt it.

I also didn't see the extent of the truly evil plan behind this work yet. I'd been posting the link to Richet's Nobel speech in every discussion on allergies or vaccine damage, hoping people would cotton on like I had. Those who listened were shocked too. When I found out about the mRNA jabs and what they were purported to do – force cells to manufacture specific proteins – the dots finally joined up to a conclusion. I brought up this conclusion when conspiracies were flying around about bio-weapons and Chinese lab leaks because I could see the giant red herring flapping around on the back of the elephant in the room.

I first proclaimed my theory in the chapter 'Proteins, Spikes and Bio-Weapons'. Few people saw it or listened so I tried again in my article 'Russian Roulette'.

I was asked to speak about this by **The Fakeologist** and

---

[116] http://vaccinetruth.org/peanut-oil.html

Spacebusters have also included it in a number of their films. [117]

Then Fakeologist sent me a long, very thorough work on the subject, best I've seen yet, 'Covid-19 Vaccines and Induced Anaphylaxis' by J.E. Lukach.

The book is full of great research but long, so I thought I'd write my own very shortened version for those with allergies to long wordy scientific articles, using my favourite KISS method (Keep It Simple Stupid)…

The author states that to his knowledge, he is the only person to recognize that anaphylaxis is the reason why "ALL mRNA VACCINES LEAVE ITS RECIPIENTS EITHER PERMANENTLY DISABLED, TERMINALLY ILL, OR IMMUNOCOMPROMISED AND SUSCEPTIBLE TO DEATH AT ANY TIME"

But he's not the only person to work this out AND he is not including all conventional vaccines in his theory, of which we KNOW the ingredients. So far we do not know the ingredients of the mRNA shots. He also seems to believe that vaccines offer 'viral immunity'. Maybe he is just being cautious here by not including the usual vaccines but why bother when anyone who speaks out about mRNA experimental gene therapy shots are being classed as 'anti-vaccine' anyway? I hope he will look further into this. (He does actually briefly at times touch on it).

He goes on to claim that vaccine manufacturers are 'infested' with eugenicists. No shit Sherlock! He also furthers that with a claim that the entire plandemic (covid) used a campaign of fear to coerce the world to take the jabs and furthering the eugenics agenda. Just like most who are only now waking up to this agenda he forgets that the exact same tactics have always been used for EVERY new vaccine campaign and its correlating 'new' disease.

But he is half right, yes, they needed a plandemic to facilitate something new. Not a vaccine though because they take at least 10 years to develop. No, they wanted an excuse to use something much more deadly (potentially) than the usual vaccines and with which they hoped to control the actual rates of death much more easily and target everyone, not just children. These shots are also not manufactured by the old vaccine manufacturers, this is a whole new conglomerate of Big pHarma and Big Tech taking a failed experimental 'treatment' for

---

[117] www.bitchute.com/channel/spacebusters/

cancer which killed all its test subjects and running with it to supposedly fight 'viruses' now.

In his book he says the side effects of the covid jabs are being 'shrugged off' as coincidence (hmmm where have we heard that before?) and that they covered their arses legally well before 2020. This was also done previously with the 1986 act giving vaccine manufacturers legal immunity from being sued if their products caused any problems. Nothing new here.

I would have to include ALL vaccines not just the mRNA which is technically not a vaccine at all but may be an even more potent anaphylaxis-inducing jab, IF their theory works and 'does what it says on the tin'.

See this guy is assuming their mRNA theory will work. I'm not so sure as I pointed out in 'The Amino Age' chapter. I think their theory is a nice cover-story for getting foreign (synthetic) proteins into our bodies. They call them 'spike proteins' and claim they are a part of their fictitious virus but they are not. They are something else but 'what?' is the question. We don't know because they will not reveal the actual contents.

Richet went on to prove that 'hypersensitivity' was an 'immune system' gone wrong, or so he thought. His work on anaphylaxis brought us more understanding of diseases which were puzzling like hay fever or asthma and how they came about. Others followed to work out why poisons/proteins from sea anemones could have the same anaphylactizing effect. Because it is injected too. What Richet showed was the process of inducing allergic reactivity and how it is permanent. The question is how many of these vaccine scientists know about this and are they deliberately trying to induce it with their vaccines?

When you understand this and people say, as someone said to me, "everyone I know has been vaccinated and they're all fine" it reminds me of this:

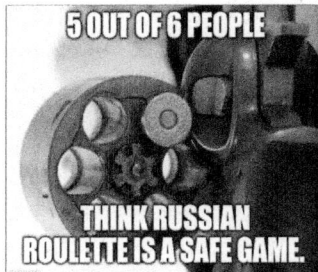

They just haven't met the full chamber yet but also they don't see their allergies or common ailments as vaccine damage because no-one has told them they are vaccine damage. "I'm fine" tends to equate to "I'm not autistic" thanks to the 'safer vaccines' campaigning of Wakefield et. al.

Richet discovered three main important factors:

1. A subject that has had a previous injection is far more sensitive than a new subject.

2. The symptoms characteristic of the second injection, such as the swift and total depression of the nervous system, do not in any way resemble the symptoms characterizing the first injection.

3. On average, a 21- day period must elapse before the anaphylactic state results. This is the period of incubation. **SOUND FAMILIAR?**

Why did Pfizer come up with a seemingly random 21 days between first dose and booster? Had they gone with 31 days, the second shot would have killed almost everyone they gave it to without emergency intervention and the campaign would have certainly screeched to a halt – like at one 'super vaccination center' in California where a few too many serious ADR's occurred. Were there a lot of already hyper-sensitised people in the line that day?

Snippet from the Pfizer-BioNTech:

Pfizer-BioNTech COVID-19 Vaccine Information CDC

CDC https://www.cdc.gov/vaccines/covid-19/info-by-product/pfizer/index.html
2-dose series separated by 21 days) A series started with COVID-19 vaccine (Pfizer) should be completed with this product.

Pfizer promptly blamed this incident on a 'bad batch' probably caused by mis-handling and lack of freezer facilities. Damage limitation spin at work. It's not our fault as always, nothing to see here. Hell it's not as if they have legal liability to worry about, as long as they can make themselves look like they're looking into it to see what went wrong and effectively putting the fox in charge of the chicken coop.

As long as no-one finds out that this is modus operandi for ALL injected proteins as according to Richet *"Instead of applying only to toxins and toxalbumins, it (anaphylaxis) holds good for all proteins whether toxic at the 1st injection or not"* (According to Wiki – "Toxalbumins are toxic plant proteins that disable ribosomes and thereby inhibit protein synthesis, producing severe cytotoxic effects in multiple organ systems). Anaphylaxis occurs after every subsequent injection, and multiple organ failure sometime thereafter.").

So do you know what you might be allergic to? Think you have no allergies? Maybe you just haven't encountered the elusive protein that was injected into you as a baby yet.

> "The anaphylactogen poison will be forever after be contained in the subject's blood."
>
> – Charles R. Richet

Now Richet adds another sinister twist to the anaphylaxis process by adding that one can be 'primed' to react by injecting someone with the blood of someone who is already primed. He discovered what he called the 'anaphylactogen' (like the word pathogen) which is a chemical substance produced by the body when primed and lingering in the blood of the anaphylactized.

I'm sure you've heard the rumour going around not to allow the jabbed to donate blood huh? Was it a rumour? Are they setting that up as a nutty conspiracy theory to be laughed at? Maybe. I'd forgo the blood transfusions though if I were you.

The thing Richet could not safely say was how long the effect of being anaphylactized lasted. If it stayed for ever or if it faded over time but he did conclude that the body never reverted back to complete normality saying "Once a subject has been anaphylactized and consequently modified in his chemical constitution, the subject can never go back to his former state. Return to normal is not possible." He did however stress that symptoms were widely varied according to the subject's constitution rather than the nature of the poison and that 'the phenomena are constant, whatever the poison used."

So there we have it. They could just prime as many people as possible then sit on it and wait for an opportune moment again to expose them to whatever they were primed with. They have all the records of who got what injected into them so they will know exactly what will work and on who. Enough time elapsing in between to point the blame at whatever they wish. It's kind of evil genius if it works.

So what is 'Anaphylactic Shock' apart from it being a severe allergic reaction?

*"The **nervous symptoms** often develop so **suddenly** and **violently** that there is no time for colic and diarrhea. **Ataxia** follows at once,"* Richet continues. (**Ataxia** describes a lack of muscle control or coordination of voluntary movements, such as walking or picking up objects. A sign of an underlying condition, **ataxia can affect various movements** and create **difficulties with speech, eye movement and swallowing.**) *"**Feelings of drunken intoxication, dilated pupils, the subject may fall to the ground, unconscious, or unresponsive. Labored or agonized breathing** is common. The **heartbeat may be faint,** there is a **rapid and acute loss of blood pressure.** All the symptoms point to the central nervous system being the seat of severe and sudden intoxication."*

This brutal assault of the poison on the nervous system is what is now called anaphylactic shock.

'Covid-19 Vaccines and Induced Anaphylaxis' by J.E. Lukach

I can think of MANY so-called diseases these symptoms could be called by modern medicine and subsequently 'treated' with pharmaceuticals. What if the whole list of new 'diseases' that have emerged since vaccines began (in the 1700's with smallpox) are actually anaphylaxis? Let's also not forget allergies were never even mentioned until the 1900's.

Among the list of more acute symptoms that Richet observed were convulsions and paralysis. Boom, we have 'epilepsy' and 'polio' right there already. I wonder how many other diseases were 'invented' on the back of this new 'reaction' to injections? One symptom could turn into a plethora of new and lucrative 'diseases' like they achieved so successfully with 'polio'.

See my article 'The CDC Issued A Vital Signs Warning Tuesday As It Prepares For A Potential Outbreak Of The 'Polio-Like Illness' in the 'Polio' chapter for more on that.

When looking for the specific ingredients that can induce an anaphylactic state Richet split them into colloids and crystalloids (colloid and crystalloid are not particles, but states of a certain substance depending on its particle size).

He said: "Crystalloids are on the whole non-active. I am not aware of any attempt to induce anaphylaxis by one crystallizable or by any alkaloid. On the other hand all the proteins, without exception, produce anaphylaxis, with all sera, milks, organic extracts whatsoever, all vegetable extracts, microbial proteinotoxins, yeast cells, dead microbial bodies. It would be of more interest now to find a protein which does not produce anaphylaxis, than to find one that does."

Proteins are the building blocks of tissues in the body which are created constantly as needed from amino acids from foods. Any alien foreign protein that is mechanically introduced is considered by the body as poison. It is that simple. Vaccines all contain antigens which are proteins. This is why they have to put 'antigens' in the vaccines to 'elicit an immune response'. All attenuated vaccines contain one or more proteins. This is what the 'attenuated viral material' is. It is just PROTEINS. The problem being – injecting the same protein more than once causes hypersensitivity; the result being – anaphylaxis. If viruses really existed and were the cause of disease why would they need to add antigens?

The more important question though has to be "do they know all this?".

Finally a bit of info on the man himself.

Professor Charles Robert Richet was a French physiologist at the Collège de France known for his pioneering work in immunology. In 1913, he won the Nobel Prize in Physiology or Medicine 'in recognition of his work on anaphylaxis'. He was also an outspoken eugenicist with a hatred of Blacks. Richet was a proponent of eugenics, advocating sterilization and marriage prohibition for those with mental disabilities. Richet expressed his eugenicist ideas in his 1919 book La Sélection Humaine. From 1920 to 1926, he presided over the French Eugenics Society. Psychologist Gustav Jahoda noted that Richet "was a firm believer in the inferiority of Blacks, comparing black people to apes, and intellectually to imbeciles."

Nice guy huh and clearly has an agenda of eugenics too. Eugenics hiding in plain sight behind white coats, research charities and labs and let's not forget the good old philanthropists like Gates and other hellth organizations wielding needles all in the name of hellth (or is it wealth?) and public policy.

Well I think that says it all really.

RUSSIAN ROULETTE

I wrote this post in 2021 for HIVE. Now that we are in the booster phase it may make a few more pennies drop to look at what I was saying back then. I've changed it and added more info and thoughts to bring it up to date…

Five months ago they were just pondering the 3rd shot.

While in the financial news there was a bit more truth to their plans:

(Reuters) -The United States is reviewing the need for a third COVID-19 booster shot among residents who have already been vaccinated but needs to see more data to know if additional shots could raise people's risk of serious side effects, a U.S. health official said Tuesday.

The official said the second dose for two-shot COVID-19 vaccine regimens was associated with higher rates of side effects, suggesting a third dose could potentially come with even greater risks.

"We're keenly interested in knowing whether or not a third dose may be associated with any higher risk of adverse reactions, particularly some of those more severe - although very rare - side effects," said Jay Butler, deputy director at the U.S. Centers for Disease Control and Prevention, during a

I've found a few of these hard hitting truth bombs always in financial articles, not in the pleb news, so hiding in plain sight.

Well what's so interesting about that you may ask? What's interesting is…they 'want to know' if a 3rd shit-shot will cause more harm than two. Seriously?

I warned about this months ago and have been warning about anaphylaxis and proteins for a while now and Richet won a bloody Nobel prize for pointing it out way back in 1913!!! You inject foreign proteins into a body once and it is primed to go crazy the next time it is encountered. You don't even have to inject it the 2nd time either if the priming is ultra-strong, take peanut 'allergies' as a prime example.

People really need to get this info absorbed and quick because you are literally being coerced into playing Russian roulette with real bullets. (5 months later it is a bit late to be warning people as most who will take it have already).

Do you know what anaphylaxis is and how it comes about though?

Phylaxis, a word seldom used, stands in the Greek for protection.

Anaphylaxis will thus stand for the opposite.

Anaphylaxis, from its Greek etymological source, therefore means that the state of an organism in which it is rendered hypersensitive, instead of being protected.

The basic premise of how to prime a body for anaphylaxis. Here are the original prize winning nasty experiments (vivisection) which exposed (or should have exposed) vaccines as a game of Russian roulette.

> An unexpected phenomenon arose, which we thought extraordinary. A dog when injected previously even with the smallest dose, say of 0.005 liquid per kilo, immediately showed serious symptoms : vomiting, blood diarrhoea, syncope, unconsciousness, asphyxia and death. This basic experiment was repeated at various times and by 1902 we were able to state three main factors which are the corner-stone of the history of anaphylaxis: (1) a subject that had a previous injection is far more sensitive than a new subject; (2) that the symptoms characteristic of the second injection, namely swift and total depression of the nervous system, do not in any way resemble the symptoms characterizing the first injection; (3) a three or four week period must elapse before the anaphylactic state results. This is the period of incubation.

Nobel prize awarded in 1913 so they knew this all since then! [118]

Then in 2021 they had the gall to post a 'new' paper pretending they had no idea about this process and giving it a new name ADE (Antibody-Dependent Enhancement). Cytokine storm was what they used to call it before covid and 'auto-immune' diseases are also a form of chronic anaphylaxis. [119]

Why are scientists pretending they knew nothing about this? It is nothing new or novel. What is new is that some of us have joined the dots and seen what they have been hiding for a long time. If you know people who have had one shot at least give them the opportunity to get off the wheel of death and not put the gun to their heads again.

(Again too late for warnings now but it does seem like the uptake of each successive shot is waning in numbers. That could also be because many died after the first shots too).

According to Richet there's a one in three chance of a bullet being in the next chamber.

I have no idea what the odds are for a third shot (and maybe neither do they which is why this is maybe a part of the grand experiment too). They are even contemplating letting the lab rats know about the bullets in the gun. [120]

Informed consent disclosure to vaccine trial subjects of risk of COVID-19 vaccines worsening clinical disease

---

[118] www.nobelprize.org/prizes/medicine/1913/richet/lecture/
[119] (www.ncbi.nlm.nih.gov/pmc/articles/PMC7943455/
[120] https://pubmed.ncbi.nlm.nih.gov/33113270/

If you take the placebo effect into account then (and GNM) knowing the risks are higher will obviously raise the numbers of reactions. (Re-read the bit about allergies and multiple personality disorders in 'Antibodies Debunked' for proof of this too).

> "Having produced antibodies against a certain substance, for example against a food or a vaccine, does not really determine whether a disease such as an infection or allergy will actually occur.
>
> For example, people with a multiple personality disorder in the role of one personality can be highly allergic to orange juice (allergen), while the same allergen, once they have switched to a different personality, suddenly no longer causes an allergic reaction One may also show symptoms of diabetes in one personality and be free of diabetes a few minutes later. Women may even have completely different menstrual cycles.
>
> Another example- In a normal person who is allergic to cat hair, when they come into contact with the proteins of cat hair, the formation of antibodies and inflammatory reactions are triggered. However, it is not uncommon for someone to be allergic only to white or red cats, but not to black cats (or vice versa). Usually there was a previous traumatic experience with a white cat – for example its death – which was related to the formation of antibodies.

So showing those who've already had the shots what could happen to them is cruel and may boost the effects and deaths rather than prevent them which is why I've steered clear of the scare stories lately. They don't help now that so many have already taken them.

It doesn't help that we are not even allowed to see the actual ingredients of these Jabberwock's either. Trade secrets!! I kid you not!! This means we have no idea what proteins might be in them so what people have been primed to react to. It's like a double blind Russian roulette with bells on.

I did point this out in 'Proteins, Spikes & Bioweapons' but it seems I need to give everyone a shake and shout a bit louder – maybe a re-read with retrospect will help?

Unless everyone gets this they can keep sending us round and round with their loaded guns (needles) until they do get their population reduction to the number they want (and five months later what are they talking about? 4th, 5th, 6th shots, shots every 3 or 6 months.

Keep shooting them till it works huh?). Or a 'booster' or who knows what else will trigger it?…

There are no 'variants'. Variants are their cover-up for the vaccine deaths and injuries. They will keep adding more variants (and more jabs) every time more reactions start occurring unless we all open our eyes to what they are doing.

As for bio-weapons which I've also touched on and debunked, who needs real bio-weapons when they already have the perfect weapon? A jab that can make you drop dead when you encounter something completely benign if you have been primed. It's like stealth bombing.

The bio-weapon, 'lab-escaped virus' and even gain of function stories are pure distractions. AND right after I posted this look what popped up in my newsfeed:

"We are seeing, right now, the highest death rate we have seen in the history of this business," Scott Davison, CEO of OneAmerica, an old and respected insurance company, recently announced. **"The data is consistent across every player in that business,"** Davison said. According to him, death claims have shot up 40 percent, primarily among people aged 18 to 64." [121]

---

[121] https://www.intellectualtakeout.org/the-unprecedented-death-spiral-of-2021/

ANTIBIOTICS

Looking down the list of recommended antibiotics on a health insurance list from 1950 there were 24 drugs listed. 70 years later (2020) we find a column of 83 different 'antibiotics'.

Back then antibiotics were described as 'novel remedies' obtained from fungi or bacteria having 'a growth-inhibiting and killing effect on pathogens'. The best known antibiotics were penicillin and streptomycin. According to the description, antibiotics are well tolerated and represent the most advanced CHEMOTHERAPY. They were hailed as miracle drugs with undreamt of curative possibilities. Still are in fact. They have since removed the word Chemo because of its connotation with cancer but chemo is what they are. The word antibiotics is made up of two words: Anti = 'against' and biotics = 'life'.

Says it all really.

Originally the 'well tolerated' bit was probably more true, but today almost all antibiotics are produced synthetically. Alexander Fleming discovered penicillin originally but it sat on a shelf for well over a decade because it killed all the guinea pigs he tested it on. Today there are different kinds of antibiotics – antibiotics that attack a specific bacterium, broad spectrum antibiotics, and so-called reserve antibiotics. These are used when nothing else 'works' due to the 'microbes' acquiring 'antibiotic resistance'. They can learn to survive.

If penicillin was administered for, say, a sore throat, it disappeared very quickly, almost miraculously it seemed. BUT it was also noted that after completing antibiotic courses most of the so-called infections simply came back. A classic example is the symptoms of scarlet fever: Here it was not uncommon for children to receive antibiotics three to five times in a row but both the rash, the fever and sore throat came back after a short time. Only when the antibiotics were dispensed with and the 'disease' finally allowed to run its course, did the symptoms completely disappear.

The fact is there is not a single antibiotic that does not cause side effects. The bacteria in the intestines that are vital for our survival, are almost always severely damaged. It can also lead to lung and nerve damage. Most of us are now aware that doctors have been prescribing far too many antibiotic drugs for many years. Today most doctors even prescribe antibiotics for so-called viral infections, knowing they are not effective because A. there are no viruses and B. viruses are not bacteria and not living.

The back story you need to understand before reading on...
Antoine Béchamp and Günter Enderlein's Findings on The Pleomorphism (Diversity) of Microbes.

Based on experiments, Béchamp developed a hypothesis called pleomorphism that has still not been refuted. According to Béchamp, all animal and plant cells consist of tiny particles, which under certain circumstances develop into bacteria and other forms. After the cell dies, these particles live on. Béchamp called these tiny particles 'microzymes' and saw that microzymes are able to replicate and have their own metabolism. They can develop into bacteria or mycelia/fungi.

According to Béchamp, the microzyme is the seed of all life. He accused the researchers of his time of only making their observations on fixed, sliced and stained, dead tissues, while his observations were of living specimens. This is still true today.

Béchamp was a contemporary of the two greatest scientific fraudsters in medical history, Louis Pasteur and Robert Koch. Béchamp accused Pasteur all his life of plagiarizing his own theories while at the same time mashing them up. In doing so, Pasteur sent medicine down the wrong (more profitable) path, which it is still on today. Pasteur rejected pleomorphism knowing that Béchamp was right, and propagated an opposing theory – monomorphism which states the shape and function of every organism is determined by its genus, species, or hereditary dispositions, which was and is complete nonsense.

Béchamp's discoveries inspired a number of scientists in the 19th and 20th centuries. The German zoologist Prof. Dr. Günther Enderlein, Wilhelm Reich and Royal Rife. Without Enderlein a special method for examining live blood, dark field microscopy, would never have been born. With a dark field microscope, one is able to see live blood to see the micro-organisms in the blood. The use of antibiotic drugs has a direct influence on the number of micro-organisms in the blood of humans, animals and even plants.

Now we've got that out of the way let's look at the two phases of dis-ease empirically proven in German New Medicine and how modern medicine is treating them so wrongly.

Most uncomfortable symptoms, as we know them, do not appear in the first phase (the sympatheticatonic phase) of what we think of as disease but GNM calls a biologically meaningful (necessary) program, but only in the second phase (the vagotonic phase) which starts immediately after the resolution of an underlying conflict.

The first phase is called the conflictive or sympathetic phase. The second phase is the healing phase or vagotonic phase. In the end there should always be a resulting normal state or 'normotonia' but only if the patient is not interfered with by physicians. Incorrect treatment often leads to the death of the patient in the first phase of a biological program. Due to the high number of cancer screening programs, many thousands of misdiagnoses are made every year and unnecessary stress triggered. In the case of breast cancer screenings, the number of women ending up with breast cancer 'diagnosis' has mushroomed in recent years which is obviously great for profits!!

In most cases patients die from over or incorrect treatment – Iatrogenesis – Death By Doctors. They will however blame aggressive cancer cells, bad bacteria or bad genes. They also claim the 'treatment' didn't work, they did everything, but the enemy, the viruses or cancer cells were just too strong, and the so-called immune system just couldn't cope. Most patients and relatives accept the word of the medical profession and usually even thank them for everything they've done.

SYMPTOMS GONE; DISEASE GONE?

The treatments – there are stimulating substances (sympathetic) such as vitamin C, taurine and caffeine, and calming substances (vagotonic) such as benzodiazepines (Valium), melatonin and morphine. Chemo drugs, including antibiotics, are stimulating (sympathetic) agents.

By giving (sympathetic) stimulating agents the patient is brought out of the (vagotonic, conflict-resolved) recovery phase, as they suppress uncomfortable symptoms. Antibiotics are really great for the relief of suffering in patients. Depending on the dosage, symptoms may disappear completely. This is the only advantage of antibiotics, the only one.

Pain disappears and so-called 'inflammation', which is very often painful, decreases. Inflammation is actually not inflammation, so not harmful, as we've all been told. The working of the microbes working in us is mistaken for 'inflammation'. The symptoms of the micro-organisms causes the tissues to be supplied with extra blood creating heat in the affected area, which can also lead to an increase in temperature in the entire organism (fever). Pain, which almost always accompanies the so-called inflammation, is caused by the water retention in the tissue without which tissue cannot be rebuilt. It is the micro-organisms that cause what we call inflammation.

So inflammation is nothing to worry about, as this is the way tissues are restored to their normal state. Administering antibiotics is like laying off the workforce rebuilding your infrastructure.

Back to GNM, in the context of 'adaptation processes' in the body, (which can also be called optimization for survival) excess tissue is broken down in the (vagotonic) recovery phase. After the conflict resolution, e.g. lung cancer – when a fear of death is over, this tissue no longer has any biological function and is broken down by the microbes until everything is as it was before the conflict occurred (to where it was before, say, a fear of death occurred). The alveoli built up during the stress phase so as to be able to breathe in more oxygen, have lost their purpose and are therefore broken down again. In this 2nd phase one feels tired and may even have a fever. The TBC mycobacteria (Mycobacterium tuberculosis), which have the task of breaking down this built-up tissue work in accord, consume energy causing fatigue and forcing us to rest. Go to bed!

Almost everyone having these symptoms, in their ignorance, will consult a physician who is also ignorant. He examines you and diagnoses tuberculosis. TB is notifiable so must be reported to the health 'authorities' immediately. During the plandemic however you would be tested for corona 'virus' and most likely immediately be told to quarantine or immediately transferred to a covid ward, where you would be connected to a ventilator. No TB patient would survive this completely inappropriate treatment. Many people worldwide die from TB mismanagement.

Best case scenario, the doctor might take blood and find that inflammation markers are elevated then prescribe antibiotics along with an antipyretic drug and send the patient home to rest. By prescribing antibiotics, the recovery phase is interrupted and regeneration prolonged. Antipyretic drugs also tend to be counterproductive. The symptoms are gone, but so is your strength. At some point the antibiotics will wear off and the body restarts the regeneration/healing phase all over again. The few micro-organisms that survived the poison attack return to work again. Ideally, they work until the breakdown of the surplus tissue is complete.

Most people are convinced we all have an immune system that can rid us of bad bacteria and viruses and even destroy cancer cells. Nobody has seen it though. In fact, there is no immune system in the way we've been sold. There are no bad microbes either, because if there were, we'd have to wonder if nature is stupid enough to put bad microbes into every living being.

We have to wonder where these microbes, which are 'evil and transmissible', are lurking in our bodies. This is important to know in the context of antibiotics. It is not the 'bad' microbes that invade us from the outside to harm us, rather, it is the inner programs that give the micro-organisms living in us their commands. Conventional medicine claims to this day that our blood is sterile which means that there are no other living organisms in the blood, but that is not true. In every drop of blood there are thousands of our friendly symbionts. These archetypes of the microbes in our blood have the ability to change their shapes, that is, their forms. The biologist Prof. Günther Enderlein (1872-1968) and earlier Antoine Béchamp (1816-1908) described this ability of the micro-organisms in our blood under the technical term pleomorphism and later Gaston Naessens filmed it.

We need microbes, the entire range of whatever is indigenous to us. If we lack these micro-organisms through overzealous 'hygiene' as in the use of chemical disinfectants, like those many were rubbing their hands with during the 'pandemic', or through the overuse of antibiotics, then the excess tissue (called tumours), cannot be dismantled in the recovery phase.

Without our little friends (symbionts, mycrozyma, protits) in the blood, it would be impossible for e.g. a thyroid carcinoma to break down the excess tissue in the recovery phase. Conventional medicine mistakenly calls this tissue a tumour. After a conflict has been resolved and without microbes, the two halves of the thyroid continue to produce thyroxine until, by encapsulation, a 'tumour' is formed. In this case, the encapsulation is called a watery cyst. This happens when the essential microbes are missing because of unnecessary antibiotic administration.

Almost every antibiotic treatment represents medical malpractice, as it can bring the bacteria, which would have broken down the 'tumour', to their knees. Of course, it is not officially considered malpractice, since orthodox doctors lack the 'universal biological knowledge' and they can only work according to the guidelines they are given, albeit absurd and counterproductive.

Mycobacteria have been around since the first protozoa appeared on earth. You might have heard the news articles claiming they've found prehistoric 'viruses' that can be 'awakened' even after millions of years. I'd humbly suggest they are looking at microzyma and not viruses though. This is why they say the world was built by these fascinating, seemingly immortal, organisms. These prehistoric creatures, the mycobacteria, are found in our bodies and can be detected in their original form in the blood. Without them we couldn't survive. They carry out the same tasks in animals as in humans. They are either used to break down excess tissue or to build it up if it makes biological sense. Skilled trauma surgeons take advantage of these skills, helping you with complicated fractures by not hermetically sealing the wound and fracture directly, but letting 'air' in. This enables and facilitates the job of the body's own 'surgeons'.

What scientists are unable to understand is why mycobacteria are so difficult to grow in the lab. Mycobacteria are grown on egg embryos. Relatively good growth can only be achieved if the living embryo used is injured in some way as a result of bad handling. As incredible as it may seem, a fear of death conflict the embryo suffers can trigger the production of mycobacteria. Mycobacteria only grow in considerable numbers if the growth is initiated by the control centre of the organism. It's really quite simple – a chicken embryo is a living being, and harm can be inflicted on any living being and tuberculosis mycobacteria only develop in the stressful phase after an injury or a fear of death, in other words, stress.

It is assumed that in the conflict-active phase the organism only lets as many acid-fast mycobacteria (rods) to develop as are needed to break down the so-called 'tumour' later, in the recovery phase, however actual research is needed to know for sure. I won't hold my breath though.

Almost all medical professionals believe that the tuberculosis bacteria are dangerous and that they have to be eradicated, fuelled by a lack of understanding of the real biological processes and intelligence of nature and the love of money and reputation.

Not only GNM but also Terrain Model says that we only actually feel unwell during a healing/detox phase. Your body is already dealing with whatever the problem is but you feel down, have a cough, sputum and suffer from night sweats and maybe a fever and that's when help is sought from a doctor. After a bunch of tests (if you're lucky) you'll be almost certainly sent home with a bunch of antibiotics, even if they're 'just in case'. The evil tubercles must be destroyed. A bit like saying all fire-fighters (bacteria) who are caught putting out fires must be executed on the spot.

Antibiotics are not curative. The only thing that happens is the symptom-laden recovery phase/healing is halted. The drugs cause you to revert to the conflict/stress phase which is when you feel fine, even quite strong. We associate being healthy with having no symptoms but are you really well? Just because you have no pain, no fever and no swelling?

For instance during the 2nd world war many people were 'scared to death' literally. The numbers of deaths from lung disease, i.e. tuberculosis or consumption, sky-rocketed during and shortly after the war. During times of war (stress and fear of imminent death) additional alveoli and mycobacteria build up in the lungs (according to GNM). When peace returned, many millions of conflicts were resolved at the same time. People switched from the conflict phase to the healing phase instantaneously. The tuberculosis mycobacteria change from the tissue building process in the lungs, which served to get more air, to degrading the tissue that was no longer needed. A prime example of how nature is constantly adapting and optimising itself. If you don't understand this, think about why muscles atrophy (waste away) when you don't use them and why muscle tissue increases when you put strains on them. Remember 'no pain, no gain'?

All microbes living in us, in their original form, are able to change their shape as soon as it becomes necessary. The commands for this come from the brain, always from the area in the brain (called relay) that is assigned to the corresponding organ. So there is a brain-organ connection. The microbes belong to us, that's clear. Dr. Hamer once said that we do not die because of microbes, but rather from the lack of them.

Most people don't understand why drugs or antibiotics seem to 'work' so well. There are only a handful of drugs that actually can help. We would be better off if 99.9% of all drugs were scrapped completely. The belief that drugs' effects are localized is false. Almost every drug works through the brain. There are few exceptions which include, for example, pain relievers ASA and ibuprofen.

Almost all drugs, including antibiotics, have an effect on the brain and thus on the control relays that signal the bacteria. Antibiotics also have a slight effect directly on the micro-organisms, because the toxic, antibiotically active ingredients are distributed throughout the body via the bloodstream. There are two main groups of drugs and natural active ingredients.

GROUP 1

Active ingredients that increase stress. These are also called 'sympathicotonics' because they stimulate the sympathetic nerve. In the stress phase, when you feel fear of death, you are in the sympathetic phase. In this phase there are no physical symptoms that would make us feel 'ill'. The best-known drugs from this group are adrenaline, noradrenaline, cortisone, hydrocortisone, chemo infusions and all 'antibiotic' substances. Natural ingredients such as caffeine are also included.

Antibiotics are nothing more than cytostatic agents that shift the body from the vagotonic recovery phase back into the stress/conflict phase. You FEEL better, but your organism is not better. Of course, it also has a direct effect on your 'symbionts', the microbes and bacteria, but only slightly. The noticeable effect comes about more because of the influence on the brain, where they cause a swelling (edema) in the correlating relay.

If you are in a symptom-heavy recovery phase, medication will help to alleviate the symptoms, because this results in a decongestion of the brain relay. At first glance, this seems desirable but it also sends the 'emergency services', our mycobacteria, back to base. The recovery phase is shut down. Any healing that was in progress is now reversed. In the best case scenario, healing may be slightly prolonged but in many cases is completely halted. In fact, sympathetic drugs, such as cortisone, are among the 0.001% of drugs that are essential, as they can alleviate the brain swelling caused by a severe healing crisis.

GROUP 2

This includes all sedatives, but also antispasmodics. They act on the vagus nerve, the resting nerve, and are therefore also referred to as vagotonic drugs. It can be used to increase vagotonia or weaken sympatheticotonia.

It is extremely dangerous to give morphine to patients who are in a severe healing crisis, in the midst of vagotonia and in pain. It is basically death by medicine. In the event of an overdose of morphine, the organism can no longer get out of the vagotonia phase. Atropine (parasympatholytic) can work as the antidote to morphine.

When antibiotics are administered, symptoms are relieved by antibiotics having a 'sympathetic' effect. The vagotonia, which manifests symptoms, is weakened. The patient feels better and the accompanying fever drops immediately. Now do you understand why antibiotics seem to work so well?

Antibiotics do not cure anything. Antibiotics should only be used in emergencies which is what they were originally classified for use as.

It was originally assumed that the bi-products of 'bad' bacteria lead to poisoning in the body and caused fever but it's not so. Today, most doctors believe this theory which has been repeated so often that it has become dogma. Out of sheer ignorance, they came up with the ingenious idea that the administration of antibiotics could prevent the tubercles producing so-called toxins through their 'breaking down' processes by destroying them before they get started. It is precisely this nonsense that doctors still believe today therefore prescribing evermore antibiotics.

It is not the poisoning from the antibiotics that leads to the decline in mycobacteria, but the action of the drugs on the brain. The mycobacteria are called back at the command of the relevant brain relay. The administration of antibiotics affects the edematized (swollen) brain region. This subsides and the symptoms become more bearable very quickly and often disappearing completely. The little tubercles immediately stop working on command. They are not killed as doctors believe either, they revert back to their microzyma phase/spore form.

The medicinal effect of antibiotics on our billions of intestinal bacteria/flora is seemingly more devastating as they revert to their dormant form and can no longer perform digestive functions causing malnutrition. Why, according to conventional medicine, are intestinal bacteria considered beneficial while other microbes in us cause 'disease'? It makes no sense if you think about it.

SUPERBUGS

Every attack on our microbes results in an archaic defensive/survival resistance on their part, hence 'superbugs' or 'multi-resistant germs'. These are not some new species of microbe at all but the same microbes in defence mode. They have simply changed tack to keep surviving and do their job. I liken it to a clean-up crew donning hazmat suits to do a dangerous job. They are defending themselves and adapting to a hostile environment but the medical experts don't see it that way and believe throwing ever more toxic poisons at them is the answer. In come the new generation of antibiotics and then even 'anti-virals'. All this to try to kill a perceived enemy which is not just 'friendly' but actually essential to life. We cannot function without them.

Before the introduction of penicillin, the streptococci ruled the hospitals, that is, they took over the clean-up work (e.g. removing 'dirt' from the wound, and actively building and breaking down cells) after injuries and operations. After the introduction of penicillin, the streptococci were replaced by the staphylococci.

With the introduction of semi-synthetically manufactured antibiotics the staphylococci were 'destroyed'. But it did not take long before the gram-positive germs were replaced by the gram-negative germs. More and more fully synthetic antibiotics (= chemotherapeutic agents) came onto the market. And again it wasn't long before a new germ called pseudomonas and with it, other 'pathogens' took over the hospital wards. It all happened about 20 years ago. Meanwhile, multi-resistant germs dominate hospitals, such as MRSA (= methicillin-resistant or multi-resistant staphylococcus aureus). If a multi-resistant germ is discovered in a patient, they immediately end up in the isolation ward.

As far as I know, there are only four reserve antibiotics in the world, which are listed as emergency antibiotics and which are supposed to be effective against MRSA. It is becoming clear that there will emerge more and more 'infectious diseases', as the germs change their form again and again because of antibiotics. However, it is not the so-called germs that will cause this, but the mistreatment by orthodox doctors who do not understand that 'germs' are in fact micro-organisms that are well-disposed towards all living things. Eventually the bacteria can become overwhelmed and no longer carry out their primary tasks of clearing up or rebuilding because the terrain is completely toxic.

Pharmacy cannot win this fight it has started. It does not end well.

The diseases of today are entirely man made. An example – if you take antibiotics, the composition of intestinal bacteria becomes skewed. Diarrhoea is a common side effect.

Another negative development and also a direct consequence of too frequent antibiotic administration is something called 'drug fever'. It is characterized by a very high fever (over 40°c) and high levels of inflammation. It is well known that antibiotics do not reduce fever and do cause 'drug fever'.

Unfortunately very few medical professionals are able to spot drug fever and its causes which are self-evident in the name and regrettably believe that more antibiotics will help.

Talk about adding fuel to the fire!! This mistake, more often than not, leads to the death of the patient.

SEPTICAEMIA

You may have noticed a recent uptick in cases of septicaemia ('blood poisoning') recently. I have. It's said to be caused by bacteria running rampant in the blood, but is it?

This old paper, entitled Chemical Versus Germ Theories of Disease by F. R. Campbell begs to differ.[122]

> 5. Suppuration will occur when there are no micro-organisms present (Orthmann). On the other hand, bacteria have been found under Lister's dressings when there was no suppuration. Paul Bert and Rosenberger have destroyed all the bacteria in a septic fluid without diminishing its septic character. Griffini has found that saliva and urine, when deprived of their micro-organisms, will produce septicæmia in rabbits, all of which facts go to prove that bacteria are not the cause of septicæmia.

suppuration = pus (infection)

A healing or detox process in the body should never be interrupted, but rather attenuated as much as possible. It is important to tinker with the symptoms as little as possible.

> you find bacteria. As an argument in favor of this view of the function of micro-organisms, we may mention the fact that in cases of septicæmia and in dead bodies the poison is most active and virulent in the earlier stages of disease or decomposition, before the bacteria are most numerous. It is upon this fact that Prof. Owen bases his theory that micro-organisms are the scavengers of the human body.

The more you turn to chemical drugs the more you lose touch with your body's workings and signals and, above all, of the actual causes of the symptoms. Symptomatic treatments are only useful in rare cases. One must identify the cause and understand the processes of the body to achieve full healing. Unfortunately, the medical system was never designed to seek, identify, and understand causes. It's not about the patient. It's about profits. It's about the sale of medicines, vaccinations and operations. Chronically ill patients bring in the most money so they will keep creating chronic illnesses (antibiotics are great for that).

---

[122] www.ncbi.nlm.nih.gov/pmc/articles/PMC9435757/?page=5

ALL ABOUT THAT MEASLES TRIAL

In 2011 Stefan Lanka (a virologist) offered a reward for proof of the measles virus. The court case was well publicised for the first part but the appeal case was blacklisted. There was nothing but crickets from the mainstream media. The reason it was blacklisted was obvious. There are many so-called 'experts' going around shouting that Lanka lost the case. They hope most people will look no further but if you do you will find that the High Court in Germany deemed the protocol used to prove any virus, the method used since 1954 by all virologists, is fraud and proves nothing. This is now case law, set in stone. The measles virus was never proven in court to exist.

Despite all the pleas of the case being only won on a technicality someone quietly took down the picture of the supposed measles virus on the online 'Big Picture Book of Viruses' (original version completely changed now). [123]

Here's the screenshot of that momentous moment again:

	paramyxovirus
	paramyxovirus
N/A	Measles virus
	Rinderpest virus
	Rinderpest virus

---

[123] www.virology.net/big_virology

Measles Virus? There Is No Proof Of A Measles Virus Says Court!

(TRANSLATED BY TRACEY NORTHERN)

(This is the article I wrote on the case back in 2017 when the appeal case was won.)

As I haven't found any English language news about the Stefan Lanka legal case, I was wondering whether you had heard about the decision of a German Court, that there was no scientific publication which proves the existence of the measles virus?

To back up – Stefan Lanka is the biologist/virologist who detected the first virus and was one of the early critics of the AIDS-HIV dogma. In 2011, he offered a €100,000 reward for anyone who presents a scientific publication that proves the existence of the measles virus and determines its diameter.

MD David Bardon presented six publications, claimed the reward and sued Lanka for refusing to pay – a first ruling had demanded that Lanka must pay. On 16th February 2016, the Oberlandesgericht Stuttgart decided on appeal, that no proof of the existence of a measles virus had been presented.

Here is a translation of an article by Hans Tolzin of Impfreport (Vaccination report), a leading website on independent vaccination education:

"Biologist Dr. Stefan Lanka does not have to pay a €100,000 reward to the Saxony based doctor David Bardens after all. Bardens had tried to prove the existence of the measles virus by submitting six publications. Lanka had offered the reward to anyone, who presented a publication, in which the virus was proven to exist and in which the diameter of the virus was determined. The District Court of Stuttgart rules in an appeal of 16th February 2016 that the demanded proof was not presented. Also the expert who was commissioned by the court, a university professor from Rostock, explicitly confirmed in the first ruling of the County Court of Ravensburg, that none of the six presented publications provided any proof of existence of the virus. Further, in explanation of the decision, the court stated that the person offering the reward also decides the conditions the bid must fulfill."

The District Court thus avoided further trouble on point. Meanwhile, several renowned university scientists support Lanka stating that science has to the present day omitted to explicitly exclude, by means of so-called negative controls, that the claimed measles viruses were in fact cell debris from cell cultures and not measles viruses.

Understandably, the verdict was a great relief for Dr. Lanka. However, the original question, whether or not there is objective evidence of a measles virus, remains unanswered so no clarity was obtained. According to the head of the court, no further clarity could be obtained by judicial proceedings.

My position (Hans Tolzin) is this – after 130 years of virology, a basic discussion was born, that was overdue. Thanks are due to Dr. Lanka, regardless of whether one believes in a measles virus or not, science can only benefit from this and so can our children, who are affected by the vaccination programs through which they claim they will eradicate the measles virus. [124]

The speaker of the court went so far as to warn journalists to be "very careful with their headlines" for the verdict does not deny the existence of the virus (it doesn't confirm it either). They insist it is only about the wording of a part of one publication, and not of all six that were presented by Bardens. The court omitted the statement from reviewers saying that not one of the publications prove the existence of the virus. The fact that six publications were presented was then left open to interpretation that maybe all of the six publications combined could prove the case, but that was never stated."

Here is Lanka's original competition text:

"The sum of €100,000 will be paid on presentation of a scientific publication, in which the existence of the measles virus is not only claimed, but actually proven, and in which the diameter of the virus is determined. The conditions of the "Infectionsschutzgesetz" (federal infection protection law) must be adhered to and therefore the publication must come from the Robert Koch Institute (German equivalent of the CDC)."

Below is a second article by Hans Tolzin with more information:

"The scientist ordered by the County Court of Ravensburg from the University of Rostock stated clearly, that none of the six presented publications on their own were capable of delivering full proof."

So far so good.

I said earlier the reviewer commissioned by the court did leave it to the interpretation of the listener to imply that all six publications

---

[124] http://www.impfkritik.de/pressespiegel/2016021701.html

combined would prove the case of the measles virus, as I found out, he gave more than a vague implication. He actually said:

"Only in overview could these (6) publications be 'regarded' as 'evidence'."

However, he didn't say they are proof, he even joked about what the definition of proof is (see below).

One reporter from Impfen-Nein-Danke.de pointed out that apparently, this would mathematically mean 6 x 0 = 6.

The text of the competition does say "One publication…that proves the measles virus." As the judge said it is not up to the justice system to decide medical facts. This can only take place in the scientific community.

It seems to me that Lanka was forced to play along with these word games to win his case.

The court got out of admitting that the existence of the virus cannot be proven by one single publication by saying it wasn't the subject of the trial to determine whether the virus exists or not. They adamantly pointed out that Lanka was only acquitted because of a small formality in the interpretation of the competition, not because the virus is not proven. As I said before they don't say the virus IS proven, either.

All in all, I see Lanka's case as an important victory in terms of challenging the paradigm of vaccination practices.

The manner in which the courts and reporters argued, somewhat reminded me of Bill Clinton saying "It depends on what your definition of the word 'is' is."

Here is a short excerpt from the transcript of the original trial of March 12, 2015 which ruled against Lanka.

At 10:55am Lanka's defendant's lawyer Schreiner addresses the scientist provided by the court, and asks to know the difference between evidence and proof.

The expert: "In biology there are only 'Indizien' (indications – circumstantial evidence)."

Lawyer Schreiner: "Could the initial measles study from 1954 be replicated using improved methods available today?"

Expert: "No, there are no sponsors/funders and no publications willing to prove this again, as it's already proven." (my comment: but he just said in biology there is only circumstantial evidence).

Scientist: "If ribosomes were found in measles virus, this would stir up attention."

Judge: "Then a need would arise for a change in paradigm, maybe a biology that works without viruses."

Scientist: "I cannot imagine a world in which virus don't exist. Publication nr. 5 is a scientific publication as well and it proves the measles virus."

(Laughter in the audience, someone shouts: "Guttenberg").

(Publication nr. 5 was one of the 6 publications cited as proof by the prosecution. It is a Journal paper that summarizes other papers without making any new findings). This goes on and on. [125]

There is another interesting detail pointed out by Kopp online in the following article, namely it seems the definition of measles virus has been changed since the announcement of the competition. In the first edition of 'Vaccine', the world's most prestigious compendium of vaccination experts, 1988, it stated: the measles virus is spherical in shape and approximately 120 to 250 nanometers in size. In the latest edition in 2013, the measles virus is not spherical any more, but can be 'various shapes'.

In addition, according to the scientist commissioned by the court, Professor Podbielski from the University of Rostock, the virus can vary in size drastically between 50 and 1000 nanometers. and lastly, another article by Hans Tolzin points out the lack of controls in the presented publications.

Solomonic verdict in measles virus trial

Hans U.P. Tolzin

"€100,000 is the sum that Biologist Dr. Stefan Lanka had promised to the person, who could present a scientific publication, in which the measles virus is proven to exist and its diameter is determined. Dr. David Bardens, a young doctor from Saarland, finally accepted this pubic challenge and he was also granted the prize money by the County Court of Ravensburg in 2015. This verdict was, to the surprise of many, overruled by the District Court of Stuttgart (OLG). The judge claims to be personally convinced of the existence of the virus but a critical condition of the bid, he decided, was not fulfilled.

With this the OLG court pulled on the emergency breaks because Lanka, in advance of the appeal trial, produced several expert assessments which pointed out, very clearly, the complete lack of control experiments in each one of the six publications presented as evidence. Such control experiments are claimed to be indispensable to

---

[125] www.impfen-nein-danke.de/wissenschaftsbetrug-heute/masernvirus-vor-gericht/

a definitive outcome of an experiment.

For instance, according to Lanka, the described experiments do not rule out that components of the cell cultures used as evidence could be erroneously claimed to be the sought virus.

According to a paper by professor Harald Walach from Frankfurt at the Oder, cited by Lanka, this is only possible using control experiments, i.e. "systematic negative controls" as Lanka called it.

A possible consequence of this statement of Walach among others could be a public dispute between scientists in court. This is something that the medical establishment wants to prevent at all costs. For where would this lead to, if suddenly some of the most important theoretical basics of the established health industry – one of the most profitable branches of industry – were publicly questioned?

The scientist ordered by the County Court of Ravensburg of the University of Rostock stated clearly that none of the six presented publications alone provided irrefutable proof, only an overview of all these publications could be 'regarded' as 'evidence'. The verdict, given by the judges, is almost a Solomonic one.

The judge personally claimed to believe in the measles virus, but the proof was to be presented in one single publication, according to the competition stipulation, and not in six different publications. Further, the head judge stated, that it is up to the person who offers the prize in a competition, to determine what conditions must be met. The judge went on to say that a court could not decide upon such scientific questions. This must happen within the scientific community. The verdict apparently came as a great relief to the defendant.

Lanka has to pay neither the €100,000 price nor the trial costs. The accuser, Dr. Bardens, has to pay the court costs.

Update: Since writing this article the MSM are still not reporting this. AND in The Picture Book of Viruses the measles virus seems to have been deleted.

After I posted my article about the measles trial I got the usual obtuse comment of it being ONLY about money. This is the ridiculous excuse Barden was giving out and all the 'sceptics' bragged about. I always laugh at their use of the word 'sceptic' as they are about as sceptical as a two year old child and this comment is just as deep. What he says though is not lying, originally it was about the prize money but that was exactly how to get this fraud really looked at, scrutinised, by the law. It might not have gone exactly as to plan but the desired effect was finally arrived at. Anyone who can't see this trial was not JUST about money is naive or plain stupid. This was a moment in medical history. There is a lot in here we can use to fight SARS/Cov2 and not only that, I feel this whole thing may have been rushed at us BECAUSE of this trial maybe before everyone knew what it actually entailed and while everyone was still claiming sour grapes and it being 'only about the money'. As Lanka said it has written history and written a new law. Now we have to use that.

From another translation I did of Lanka's article on the whole measles trial – 'All About That Measles Trial' (original in German): [126]

As of December 1, 2016, the highest court ruling in Germany stipulates that all claims regarding the infection called measles, measles vaccinations and the measles virus have no scientific basis.

The reasons for the judgment, confirmed by the highest court, include clear statements of fact that refute not only all claims regarding the infection of measles, measles vaccinations and the measles virus, but also all so-called 'disease-causing viruses' and vaccinations. Now the world waits for the first court case in which this supreme court ruling can be used, in which a compulsory vaccination, an exclusion from school, an encroachment on parental rights or the right to free choice of profession, the recognition of vaccine damage or the untenability of the state vaccination recommendations is challenged.

This can and should lead (first in Germany and then globally) to an admission of undesirable developments in medicine and to the beginning of a truly scientific, public health education system. The foundations for this have been laid.

(The naysayers also complain about the 6 papers submitted being evidence of a measles virus if you take them in combination. Lanka's and the courts answer to this complaint is pretty conclusive though).

Under paragraph 122 of the judgment, the OLG came to the conclusion that my appeal was successful because proof of the existence of the measles virus through 'a scientific publication' was not fulfilled by the plaintiff. The court referred to the court-appointed expert, Prof. Podbielski, who testified in writing before the first court and orally stated that none of the six publications offered by Dr. Bardens contained evidence of the existence of the 'measles virus'.

Prof. Podbielski's construct of turning six non-proofs into one

---

[126] www.northerntracey213875959.wordpress.com/2021/10/28/all-about-that-measles-trial/

scientific proof, which the Ravensburg Regional Court followed, was rejected by the appellate court. Thus it was judicially determined and is now German case law, which can no longer be disputed, that none of the six publications contain evidence of the existence of the 'measles virus'.

What is significant about the OLG/BGH jurisprudence on the 'measles virus' is that today all 'disease-causing viruses' are 'proven' with the method invented by Enders in 1954. This method, which Enders described in mid-1954 as speculation "to be regarded with extreme caution", became a 'scientific fact' when Enders was awarded the Nobel Prize on 10 December 1954 and became the model and standard for all current methods of detecting 'pathogenic viruses'.

On February 16, 2016, the Stuttgart Higher Regional Court not only wrote world history on the 'measles virus', but also refuted the 'scientific nature' of claiming the existence of any 'disease-causing viruses' and the effectiveness of the 'protective' vaccinations.

From the announcement of the legal validity of the Stuttgart OLG judgment of February 16, 2016 by the Federal Court of Justice on December 1, 2016, all 'measles vaccinations' and coercive measures regarding them are illegal. Measles vaccinations per se and all related restrictive measures are forbidden from December 1 dn[st], 2016, since they are no longer justifiable but criminally prosecutable infringements on the basic rights to physical integrity and life, education, parental rights and free choice of profession.

As a result of the inquiries relating to the measles virus: The RKI had internal studies on the 'measles virus', but contrary to the clear obligation of the RKI to publish all examinations, they were not published.

The reason for the refusal of the RKI to carry out and publish studies on the 'measles virus' became clear through their own admission on January 24, 2012. This document refutes claims that the 'measles virus' exists as well as claims that measles vaccination is safe and effective. The RKI writes in it:

"Like other paramyxoviruses, measles viruses do not show a precise size or a precise diameter: they measure from $120 - 400$ nm in diameter and then often also contain ribosomes inside. 'Ribosomes' are the cell's own factories with which humans, animals and plants produce proteins." Since the 'measles virus' cannot possibly contain any 'ribosomes', this admission by the RKI refutes all claims of the existence of the measles virus! Even more – The RKI has admitted that it works with normal components of life and cells not "measles viruses". Even more, the RKI has thus provided proof of why the measles vaccination in particular, above all other standard vaccinations, generates the highest rate of vaccine damage in the form of allergies and autoimmune reactions.

The auxiliary substances contained in all vaccines (so-called adjuvants, in reality potent neurotoxins) are supposed to stimulate immune reactions against the alleged viruses. Indeed, the body develops immune reactions, but instead of the alleged helpful reactions, allergic 'auto' immune reactions against itself, because with a measles vaccination typical endogenous proteins are implanted instead of a 'foreign' body.

In section 117 of its judgment of February 16, 2016, the OLG Stuttgart announces the refutation of the entirety of virology by their expert. The reviewer is quoted as saying: "The conceptual understanding of the virus is in fact in a state of flux." What Prof. Podbielski kept secret is the fact that well-known 'virologists' are again changing and redefining the whole of virology, just as they did back in 1951 and 1952. They have recognised that structures that were misinterpreted as 'viruses' are themselves alive and our cell nuclei emerge from them. They advocate that these structures be recognised as a fourth classification of life alongside the previously discovered 'kingdoms' of life, the primordial bacteria, the bacteria and the true cells, and be designated as such. As a young student I was lucky enough to be the first to isolate such a harmless structure from the sea, to fully characterize it and of course (along with control experiments) to publish it scientifically.

Now it gets even MORE interesting…

In 1997 the world's greatest scientific fraud so far became public. All data relating to the existence of a 'hepatitis B virus' and a vaccination against cancer, involving hundreds of the most prominent AIDS, gene, immune, infectious disease and cancer scientists, were not only falsified, but fictitious. As a result, public prosecutors, parliamentarians and politicians demanded that scientific fraud be made a criminal offense.

The German Research Society (DFG), an association that distributes billions in research funds on behalf of the government, called on politicians not to introduce the planned criminal offense of 'scientific fraud'. The DFG claimed that science should control itself. (Pfffff). In Germany, since 1998, all scientists and institutions that receive state research funding have been obliged to adhere to this ingenious, logical and simple set of rules in their work and in the preparation of reports.

The following is central to every newly introduced method that is supposed to produce scientific knowledge: "Control experiments with complete disclosure of the experimental set-up are a central part of the scientific methodology in order to verify the methods used and to exclude disruptive factors."

Publications without documented execution of control tests may not be presented as scientific. (I wonder if this applies worldwide?)

Final word on the '6 papers to be used in conjunction' complaint –

The plaintiff, the Homburg MD Dr. Bardens now works in Sweden. As an explanation for having lost the case brought by him at the Stuttgart Higher Regional Court and the Federal Supreme Court in Karlsruhe, he presented an explanation to the media which he freely invented. He claims that he lost due to a technicality. Dr. Bardens claims that he lost because instead of submitting one publication he submitted six publications.

Nothing like this can be found in the oral hearing before the OLG Stuttgart and in the written grounds for the judgment. On the contrary. Dr. Bardens lost the trial because the court-appointed expert found that none of the six publications presented contained evidence of the existence of a virus. That was also the only true statement of the expert, Prof. Podbielski. The argument of Prof. Podbielski, "the statements of combinations of the 6 publications are necessary for the evidence (of the measles virus)", was expressly rejected by the OLG Stuttgart.

WHAT IS DISEASE?
ANSWER FROM A DEAD NURSE

**"There are no specific diseases, only specific conditions"
– Florence Nightingale**

When I first heard this quote from the great nurse I wasn't quite sure what it meant. It is not amongst the most famous of her quotes as it flies over most peoples' heads but it is probably the most dangerous of her quotes to the medical establishment if everyone understood what it means. I will try to explain.

A while back I was discussing what to write next after my 'germ theory trilogy' and it came to mind that we need to understand what 'disease' actually is and also what it is not.

Pre-modern medicine there were few named diseases. The plague and the Black Death were the two generic names for mass disease and death spanning 400 years or so it goes. Then we had the pox which included leprosy and syphilis, then smallpox and then many other new-fangled labels started appearing.

Germ theory gave them a perfect new bogeyman.

I posted this about five years ago: **"The whole aim of practical politics is to keep the populace alarmed – and hence clamorous to be led to safety – by menacing it with an endless series of hobgoblins, all of them imaginary" – H.L. Mencken**

I would liken the named diseases we have now, and there are thousands, with more being added by the day, to a kind of 'branding'. In marketing the brand is all important for selling and making big money.

Everything has to be branded these days. Once you have a brand you can market it, produce products for it, then build charities and companies with it to create more income. Then you can target your market and recruit more customers with 'awareness campaigns' and 'screening' but the jackpot for every brand is its very own patented drug, protocol, procedure or vaccine. Once the vaccine or drug is out there it will in itself create more new 'diseases' to name/brand and market.

Hell they even have a market for recycled organs from unfortunate not quite dead people to stuff into others who've had their organs whipped out when they've damaged them beyond their scope of repair (or so they claim).

How many of these brands do we have out there now? According to the CDC website just under 'A' there are 52 or thereabouts. [127]

Many of these brand names are long winded and Latin so for ease of marketing they've taken to initializing and coming up with catchy acronyms like ALS, AIDS, ADHD and on and on…

If the anachronism isn't catchy enough they'll use old fashioned scare names like Mad Cow Disease or shorten a long name like Ebola Virus Disease to a more catchy, simple, Ebola. Something which will stick in your mind, or as they like to say in marketing 'resonate with you'. Once you have your brand, according to a 'brand strategy' website I looked at, you can:

1. Attract cult-like following

2. Makes more sales

3. Grows faster

4. Get better ROI

(ROI = return on investment). [128]

All this naming and 'branding' of 'specific diseases', as Florence calls them, is a way of redefining variations of a few symptoms into a marketable product.

It's a money-making scam. They would have us believe all these diseases are only just now being discovered through 'science' but is that true? According to Florence, no, "there are no specific diseases."

Now I know you're going to complain that she was working in the field before modern medicine and its technology were even invented therefore she would be proven wrong in the future. But actually she was dead right and if she was alive today she'd soon be dead.

Modern medicine first tried to pin their 'specific diseases' each on a specific germ/microbe which Florence completely rejected before Pasteur got his hands on the theory and promoted it with (or rather

---

[127] https://www.cdc.gov/DiseasesConditions/az/a.html

[128] https://www.ebaqdesign.com/blog/brand-strategy-elements

because of) Rothschilds/Rockefellers backing.

If you look up her thoughts on germ theory you will get a load of websites which claim she came around in the end to believe in the notion of germ theory but those claims are also false. To put the quote above into context and explain her thinking you need to look at the whole piece it came from:

"Diseases are not individuals arranged in classes, like cats and dogs, but conditions growing out of one another. Is it not living in a continual mistake to look upon diseases as we do now, as separate entities, which must exist, like cats and dogs, instead of looking upon them as conditions, like a dirty and a clean condition, and just as much under our control; or rather as the reactions of kindly nature, against the conditions in which we have placed ourselves?

I was brought up to believe that smallpox, for instance, was a thing of which there was once a first specimen in the world, which went on propagating itself, in a perpetual chain of descent, just as there was a first dog, (or a first pair of dogs) and that smallpox would not begin itself, any more than a new dog would begin without there having been a parent dog.

Since then I have seen with my own eyes and smelled with my own nose smallpox growing up in first specimens, either in closed rooms or in overcrowded wards, where it could not by any possibility have been 'caught', but must have begun. I have seen diseases begin, grow up, and pass into one another. Now, dogs do not pass into cats. I have seen, for instance, with a little overcrowding, continued fever grow up; and with a little more, typhoid fever; and with a little more, typhus, and all in the same ward or hut.

Would it not be far better, truer, and more practical, if we looked upon disease in this light (for diseases, as all experience shows, are adjectives, not noun-substantives). True nursing ignores infection, except to prevent it. Cleanliness and fresh air from open windows, with unremitting attention to the patient, are the only defense a true nurse either asks or needs.

Wise and humane management of the patient is the best safeguard against infection. The greater part of nursing consists of preserving cleanliness. The specific disease doctrine is the grand refuge of weak, uncultured, unstable minds, such as now

rule in the medical profession. There are no specific diseases; there are specific disease conditions."

From this we can see she did not believe that all these new named diseases were separate entities at all. They were and are just variations of symptoms of the only three actual causes of sickness. She saw and believed that sickness was caused by environment (the word used in its broadest meaning). She followed the theory put forward by the 'natural hygiene' proponents. The word hygiene has also since been usurped by modern medicine to mean 'killing germs' when it meant actually clean living as in fresh air, fresh food and a positive attitude/clean thoughts. The word hygiene back then had no link to germs whatsoever. In fact we now know that bacteria are in abundance in fresh fruit and vegetables as they are in our own bodies. All processing including cooking kills the bacteria hence the difficulty in digesting it. Bacteria ARE the digesters. Everyone and everything living has its own microbiome which break down dead cells into their recyclable parts – the amino acids. Without the bacteria in the living food you eat you may as well eat rocks. If you still believe the stomach digests food in 'acid' then you might like to read Robert O'Young's new explanation of how the stomach really works.

But I've digressed a little, let's get back to those diseases.

What is disease? In general it is a dis-ease. Something is not running smoothly any more. It is a spanner in the works if you want to continue thinking materialistically. It could be a lack of oil in your engine. The wrong fuel or maybe a wire has come loose.

Let's take a cough as an example. Have you ever accidentally had something 'go down the wrong way', you're drinking and something shocks you into breathing so liquid goes down the pipe to your lungs. I've done it a few times and it is awful, you feel like you can't breathe in as your body will only exhale, a horrible coughing fit until you're blue in the face. This is your amazing defense system working to prevent liquid from getting into your lungs and drowning you.

Would you call that a disease, give it a marketable name? No, because you know why it happens and the reason for it. The same process is triggered if too much dust is inhaled and even poisonous chemicals. This is your 'immune system' and its 'symptoms' doing its thing, expelling stuff which could kill you by clogging everything up or killing your cells/tissues/organs. This is what 'hygiene' tries to prevent.

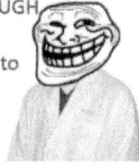

If You have a Bad COUGH,
Take LAXATIVES
Then you'll Be Afraid to
Cough

A joke yes, but too close to the truth of modern medicine.

Same thing applies to vomiting, in a way, in that the body will immediately eject what it does not want or cannot digest. There don't seem to be any specific diseases based on vomiting alone though, obviously not easily marketed apart from the old Thalidomide disaster to supposedly prevent morning sickness in pregnancy.

It turns out morning sickness is only our body's way of keeping out bad food and putting in what the body needs and making it bloody obvious what it wants and what you should avoid.

This is obviously more crucial to a foetus full of dividing cells which is when they are most vulnerable to permanent damage.

The old saying 'listen to your gut' springs to mind. While pregnancy is still not a disease, there is no lack of trying to make it one. They tried to outlaw midwives back in the early 1900's from practicing in America (within the system). [129]

And how many babies are born outside of the clinical modern medicine setting of hospitals these days? Not many and mostly by accident.

Skin diseases showing themselves with rashes, poxes and even boils are again the body expelling poisons or waste products through the holes (pores) in your largest organ of the body. Yes your skin is classed as an organ and it is not an impermeable barrier as many would believe. What you put on your skin gets absorbed but if it is poisonous it will be ejected too. Your skin is the first line of defense from all kinds of pollutants. All those chemical cleansers you smother on your face and body, the chemicals you wash your clothes in can be ejected right back out IF the pores are not blocked with dirt or oil that is (think blackheads). Depending on the kind of pollutant and the severity of exposure the symptoms will differ from a bit of itching to massive pustules named smallpox. I wonder why they called it 'SMALLpox at

---

[129] www.statnews.com/2022/10/12/maternity-care-in-the-u-s-is-in-crisis-its-time-to-call-the-midwife/

the time. Was there ever a BIGpox? Remember that 'hygiene' again, clean clothes and skin means washing away those pollutants, not smothering your pores with oily creams and such. Clean water and maybe a simple pure soap is all that's needed to wash the skin clean of harmful pollutants if you've been exposed to them and to let them back out if they get in.

I could go on to list other symptoms which would make this too long and complicated; suffice to say if the original expelling symptoms are stopped or quashed (which is all that modern medicine seeks to do ultimately) the damage from the pollutants will go deeper, to the organs where they never would have arrived at if you'd listened to your gut, if you get my drift. All the major signs your body is detoxing something, put together will come under most acute disease symptoms and they all begin with the same short list of coughing, sickness, mucus, temperature which put you in the brand name specific diseases of a flu or a cold. ALL diseases start with the same symptoms, look it up, therefore the next phase, if whatever it is being detoxed is blocked by their treatments, will be more intense and be given a new name and brand even though it is the same exact cause and process. Remember those dogs and cats…

The goal of modern medicine is to prevent our body's innate defense systems from doing their job of expelling, creating deeper and more damaging effects inside the body, therefore creating their new and unnatural 'specific diseases' with marketing names and branding. All their drugs are just poisons with brilliant marketing. Allowing those poisons to get through to the organs will put your body into shock. When your body is in shock you will not feel any of the original and obvious symptoms, which although not pleasant are absolutely necessary to protect your organs. So while you may feel better you are actually much more sick, you just don't know it yet.

The next phase of the body's attempt to fix this situation will be again named and marketed with a new brand of disease to be rinsed for all its worth. For example a cough gets suppressed with a new drug, the lungs become clogged with the stuff your cough was trying to expel and you have bronchitis, the cough is again suppressed, the mucus built around the offending pollutants does not get coughed up either and you end up with trouble breathing, asthma, pneumonia all the things the body was trying to prevent of damage to the lung tissues. What we see and feel are worse symptoms trying to prevent the organ failure and death. Inflammation is NOT caused by the body, it is caused by the poisons in the body where they shouldn't have reached, injuring the tissues and cells there. Damaged and dead cells have to be cleaned out ASAP.

Using an as above so below analogy, look what happens if the garbage men don't come around and clean the streets, the rats move in to clean up the mess. So it is in the body, garbage has to be dealt with or it will build up and create a polluted environment meaning the big boys have to get in there too. These would be the bacteria always seen at this scenario and blamed for the original mess. The old flies and garbage analogy – the flies do not create the garbage. The only way to cause diseased organs is to prevent the body protecting them with those excretory pathways or to bypass the excretory system altogether by injecting poisons straight into the body proper. Vaccines have been one of the greatest weapons used against us for this reason. You cannot cough, spew or shit that stuff out once it is in your body. You are in deep trouble. The walls have been breached using a Trojan Horse.

No-one needs a PHD or doctor's qualification to understand disease, in fact they are just pieces of paper to certify that the owner has read and understood the fairy-tale nonsense they have concocted on the foundations of germ theory. All their flowery, 'Latiny', 'sciencey' language is just a magical veil of mystery to cover up the original lie that has been blown out of all proportion. Remember, a good liar has to have a very good memory. It's all a big cover up. None of it is right and none of their learning will help you get permanent relief. Your body is perfectly designed to be healthy and to live to 120. All remote populations who never see a doctor live to over 100 and not as bed-bound vegetables with no quality of life either. The common denominator in all the longest living healthy populations are remoteness from 'civilization', clean living and most importantly a lack of medical doctors. So now you know what dis-ease is and is not, what are the causes, or as Florence calls them 'disease conditions', apart from the obvious already outlined above? My personal list is very short:

> "There are only three diseases: toxemia, malnutrition, and injury (physical or mental)." ~ Tracey Northern

Just to make it clearer I can break down this short list of 3 for you:

TOXAEMIA – Poisoning by various methods, eating it, drinking it, breathing it in, rubbing it in through the skin, most of which can be dealt with by the body if it is allowed to. Injected poisons is another matter which could be described as deep or organ poisoning. Even their one supposed miracle of modern medicine – antibiotics are just poisons. Anything which purports to kill bacteria is going to kill your own cells much quicker because bacteria have their own defense mechanism.

Antibiotics don't kill them, they cause them to change (morph). Look up 'pleomorphism' which is well known in science but not taught to us plebs. Germs/bacteria can and do change shape and function according to their environment.

Fungus is not separate from bacteria, it IS bacteria in another form, in fact the form they adapt to for the most toxic circumstances – like an assault of antibiotics. This is why you will see 'thrush' after a course of antibiotics. It's your own bacteria being 'undead'.

If you want to learn more about this germ theory debunking morphing Gunther Enderlein is your man and now more recently Gaston Naessens. [130]

If your blood becomes toxic (brand name 'sepsis') you will have a lot of dead and dying (poisoned) blood cells. A dead blood cell no longer carries a charge, the thing that keeps them all repelled from each other like little magnets repel. Once dead or dying they clump into brand name 'Thrombi' – thrombosis, erm Covid-19 or the 'delta variant'. Some more new brand names for you.

MALNUTRITION – No I'm not talking about a lack of calories either. Malnutrition is eating the wrong foods/wrong diet (BAD nutrition) and being depleted in nutrients. Remember scurvy? A lack of fruit caused horrific disease and ultimately death and if you think it was cured or abolished take a look around you. Scurvy is all around us in people who do not eat fresh fruit and vegetables. Just look up the symptoms of scurvy if you don't believe me. Rotten teeth is one of the first visible signs so why are dentists now telling their trusting customers that fruit rots your teeth?!! Quacks the lot of them! Dairy was always hailed as building strong bones by medical doctors but it's

---

[130] www.life-enthusiast.com/articles/pleomorphism-gunther-enderlein/
www.life-enthusiast.com/articles/pleomorphism-gaston-naessens/

been found that dairy actually leeches nutrients FROM the body, specifically calcium which the body uses to buffer the acids created to digest the complex proteins in it. So exactly the opposite is the case, the loss of calcium leads to weaker bones, brand name: 'Osteoporosis', a named disease found only in heavy dairy eating countries.

Drugs can also cause malnutrition as it takes a lot of certain amino acids and proteins/enzymes in the body to neutralize the poisons. Here you can find a comprehensive list of nutrient depletion caused by drugs. [131]

INJURY (PHYSICAL OR MENTAL) – OK the first bit is obvious, a physical injury causes dis-ease of course but what about the mental aspect? We know the mind can affect the body, that's obvious too although many still refuse to believe even that. Hello, placebo effect anyone? Placebo effect is so well recognized it is actually always supposed to be included in any scientific research of drugs. It is also well known that one can die from a sudden shock if the body is not kept warm and given some sugar (emergency and easily absorbed energy). This is simply explained, the body/mind's survival was threatened, the sugar is instant food and the warmth gives a feeling of safety and shelter therefore the threat is over. If you are not open to the possibility of the mind causing physical sickness in the rest of the body then you may as well stop reading now and go play Pokémon.

If you are open then I suggest you take a hard look at German New Medicine which has been empirically proven and verified. Certain shocks to the psyche produce a survival mechanism in the body which modern medicine has perceived as diseases – many, many different specific named and branded diseases. Learning GNM will save you a lot of grief and poisoning to death by the medical protocols they have assigned to some of these healing processes. I am not one to focus everything on one paradigm though and don't believe every disease is caused by a shock, the ones that are can easily be verified by a brain scan where the GNM shock can be clearly seen. These lesions have been misinterpreted as brain tumours by modern medicine.

Last but not least there is the realm of energy, our body's electrical

---

[131] www.steadyhealth.com/articles/are-the-drugs-you-take-making-you-lose-essential-vitamins-and-minerals/specific-drugs-and-the-nutrients-they-deplete

system which if 'injured' can cause havoc in the body. Think blowing a fuse or tripping a wire. In the case of autism and maybe epilepsy the wires have been stripped of their insulation causing short circuits and cross connections. The body's energy field is relatively unchartered territory in the mainstream despite them using electricity on the brain and heart in emergency cases to 'reset' things. The heart producing its own currents ties in with Tom Cowan's new theory of the heart not pumping at all but producing a vortex. They know that blood cells carry a small negative charge. How else do you think they do not clump together until the charge is lost when they are dead?

Lots of people are looking into this aspect of health now. I am only learning properly about it now and just bought my first tuning fork. When my son was young and suffering from asthma attacks after a diphtheria vaccine was shoved down his throat, I took him to alternative practitioners who used reflexology and a machine which had a bunch of crystals in a wand attached to it. I had no idea how it worked but it surely did. This was energy medicine as written about by Raymond Rife and Wilhelm Reich. [132]

Of course their work is heavily censored and as I always say, if they don't want us looking at it, it must be damned-well worth looking at. I use the analogy of electricity as it is easiest to understand but the body's energy system is more than just electrical, that is only one form of energy we can perceive. There are many other frequencies more difficult to mentally understand or see. Think OM. Think Chinese Chi. Then there are radio waves and beyond…remember where I said near the beginning the words 'resonate with you'? I think they know more than they are letting on. Maybe their Trojan Horse poisons can only resonate with a body already in a certain frequency? That's how resonance works. Fear is a frequency or it changes the frequency of the body making it more susceptible to illness by resonance. That is another theory which makes more sense than the old germ one. We are now entering into the metaphysical realm where science dares not tread for fear of the curse of 'woo'. [133]

Onwards into the unknown and the unknowable…

---

[132] www.thoughtco.com/wilhelm-reich-and-orgone-accumulator-1992351
www.royal-rife.com/

[133] www.nutritionalbalancing.org/center/environment/articles/emf-emr-health-effects.php

There is no easy to find proof of the injuries being caused by EMF's and this new 5G but you can bet it is a major cause of the mass illness and hysteria going on now. Plenty of proof in the free e-book called The Invisible Rainbow. [134]

There is no way they can let it be known that their new waves might injure us so they invented a new virus and a new disease to scapegoat any of the many possible symptoms when they started switching it on. They even had their branding and products all ready to go with this one as if they knew when and where the trouble would start. (Wuhan was the first trial of the 'internet of things'). What an amazing job they've done in hoodwinking the whole world, those who weren't hoodwinked may still be 'made dead' soon like the three African leaders who all conveniently dropped dead suddenly after refusing the marketed 'vaccines'. This has to be the biggest marketing ploy in the history of snake-oil sales to date.

IN SHORT – To summarize, all diseases are originally a healing process in the body. Yeh it may be unpleasant for a while but then who enjoys cleaning a cesspit? Who said it will be good clean fun? Always remember no pain, no gain…no gain and you're on the scrapheap. Your body and its microbes are not out to kill you and their symptoms are not harming you either. The 'treatments' on the other hand can and do kill.

IN A NUTSHELL – Modern medicine and its extensive, ever-growing arsenal of poisons and pharmakeia are producing most of the new dis-eases which they will happily inflict on anyone who willingly offers themselves up to their quackery.

Modern medicine has also always produced the scapegoats to cover up for diseases caused by environmental poisons pumped out by big industries coincidentally also owned by the same people who own big pharma and now big tech. EMF's are possibly to be a new and more deadly 'pollution' Stop being deceived. As they preached to us about the other drugs not officially in their marketing scheme – Just Say No.

Addendum

I've had some comments claiming Nightingale never said the words I've used in this article. I have two proofs she did. One is from another book – How to Live and Eat for Health by P. L. Clark, M.D. in which

---

[134] www.researchgate.net/publication/330287405_The_Invisible_Rain bow_A_History_of_Electricity_and_Life

he quotes Nightingale in full from her book Notes on Nursing.

The second proof comes from my friend Jim Dandy who said this:

> **Jim Dandy**
> **Tracey Northern** I would have said to the naysayers to provide proof. I had 2 books by her called Notes on Nursing. The first earlier one had it in the first few pages. The second one written much later did not have it. I am sure that the medical mafia backed by phama did not wont nurses in traing to have access to that information. Plus this man who wrote about it in 1935. I don't think he just made it up. He really didn't need Nightingales comment to make his point.

More proof that the truth is being censored. There is a limit to how much we can prove in this fight so please use your own discernment in future.

*There's also an audio version of this article on Odysee – with thanks to Fakeologist * [135]

---

[135] https://odysee.com/@northerntracey:a/Let's-Go-Branding_mp4_Low_:2

THE FUTURE OF MEDICINE

I've mentioned German New Medicine a few times but now it's time to take a closer look at where it stands now and going forward, hopefully with a better way of taking care of the sick than what we've all just been intensively subjected to in the last few years.

I won't be explaining the details of GNM yet.

A. because I do not know the intricate details and B. I am not qualified to teach them (this will be important later in this piece.)

Many people are starting to hear about GNM now and with Lanka's public seal of approval it feels like the time is right to lay all the cards on the table and work out how we move forward.

Modern medicine has kind of hit a wall over the last three years. Many people have seen the cracks now and how big they actually are. It has kept us all in its claws using fear. Fear of illness, what it's about, the scary treatments and suffering to impending death if we don't comply. The culprit allegedly being our own bodies, badly designed and out to kill us at every turn it seems. If it ain't the dreaded germs and viruses that'll beat you it's your very own body that will.

That's about the gist of it anyway.

The only thing so far that we've been told can save us from ourselves and the bogeymen are those knights in white cotton overcoats. The mercury wielding pharmakeia merchants. Their story hasn't changed over the last 200 years, it has just evolved lots more bells and whistles, tinsel and baubles. Any alternatives to 'modern medicine' have been relegated to the 'Woo' cupboard for hippies and crystal collectors plus the desperate injured rejects released back to nature to die of their inflicted medical injuries.

Some of us are left wondering if they simply overstepped the mark with this silly pandemic ruse. Most of the new money-spinner drugs seemed to be anti-viral drugs so were they trying to boost sales? Fuel the fear factor a bit more? Could be. The anti-virals were a bit of a Catch-22 for them though as they could take away from vaccine sales (if either of them worked, lol).

Anti-vaxxers were on to their game and sales were plummeting pre-covid. They needed a boost too, not competition.

BUT we saw the dancing doctors and nurses while being told they were 'overwhelmed'. We heard the stories that just didn't gel of a new deadly virus and disease. Then we learned they had no virus, the vaccines weren't vaccines, the figures weren't adding up. Let's not forget the old 'Doctors are baffled' along with the 'baffled' scientists too. Not to mention the very sick and twisted treatment of our elderly, locked away and murdered with death row drugs and starvation. Suffice to say a lot of respect has been lost and replaced with mistrust and anger.

Can they pull off a reinvention of modern medicine with their merger with nanotechnology? That depends on us.

Healing started out as an art, a gift. Then we had the herbalists all killed off by the church under the guise of witch hunts. Then they took the herbs and merged with big chem to bring us Rockefeller medicine. Now that is to merge with Big Tech while the suffering sick people have become nothing more than statistics, data and lab rats.

So what do we do now?

We could see an emerging new outlook. Many are looking into 'terrain theory' and many are now preaching of new paradigms and methods. But are they preaching facts or putting their own slant on old methodologies? They've certainly dusted off the old 'Hygienists' but they seem to be taking a giant black marker to their writings too. Terrain theory is not just about environmental issues, it's also about diet. Look up their methods for yourself and see what they recommended to keep your body 'clean'. Dr. Herbert Shelton is the most prominent teacher of 'natural hygiene' but most of the emerging voices are not sticking to his tried and tested methods. TC Fry was another, so all those saying I have an agenda over diet, no it's you who have an agenda and want to change or ignore the original teachings of terrain theory, not I.

There's an interesting but, as always, biased history of natural hygiene on Wiki. [136]

Never before in the history of wellness has eating dead animals been recommended for a healthy body/terrain until the last 50 years maybe and definitely pushed even more in the last 20. Now the vegans are even being blamed for agenda 2030 or being mocked as 'victims' of propaganda. I think the word mirroring springs to mind (or is it projection?) who cares.

What seems to be happening is these new-age ex doctors are taking the hygienists teachings and moulding them into something more 'palatable' for the 'chicken-soup' loving truther community as they see

---

[136] https://en.wikipedia.org/wiki/Orthopathy

them. A case of the blind leading the blind? No, something worse.

Apart from terrain theory/natural hygiene what else do we have? Energy medicine, chakra's and tuning forks. All possible aids maybe but do they actually cure? Nothing is proven 'scientifically' but no surprises there. There's no money in Big pHarma verifying their opponents and they still hold all the money and regulatory power, besides the body heals itself IF we let it.

Another less-known 'bandwagon' that's been hovering in the wings is called German New Medicine (or just New Medicine). It is definitely new by modern standards as it was discovered in the 80's by a German doctor. Dr. Hamer was an Internist and a Dr. of Theology who worked with cancer patients.

The Wiki intro to Hamer is hilarious:

"Ryke Geerd Hamer (17 May 1935 – 02 July 2017) was a German ex-physician and the originator of Germanic New Medicine (GNM), also formerly known as German New Medicine and New Medicine, a system of pseudo-medicine that purports to be able to cure cancer. The Swiss Cancer League described Hamer's approach as 'dangerous, especially as it lulls the patients into a false sense of security, so that they are deprived of other effective treatments."

They give the game away that this was written with a mouthful of 'sour grapes' with their first ridiculous claim of him being an 'ex-physician'. You can't be an ex anything before having been that thing previously. It also gives the game away as to when it was written. So he was in fact a PHYSICIAN. Yes he was struck off obviously, the same goes for anyone who dares to question the modern medicine modality. Toe the line or get out (Wakefielded).

Wiki also explains Hamer's Iron Rules quite well and accurately from what I can see but they seem to have added an addendum at the end of them.

"Hamer. These 'laws' are dogmas of GNM, not laws of nature or medicine, and are at odds with scientific understanding of human physiology."

They had to get a little dig in there at the end, lol. How ingenious. Hamer certainly was 'at odds' with modern medicine dogma for sure. You have to love their projection of their own 'dogma' onto the anti-dogma of GNM.

Moving on, it's not scientific to attack using ad hominem but they have to because Hamer's work IS scientific. He developed it while working in oncology and universities, by collecting empirical data and brain scans of his sick patients (not lab rats) and even learning from his own cancer diagnosis. He ticked ALL the scientific, empirical, methodical boxes in his work but it was the results the establishment were not happy with for very obvious reasons.

The two main things they are not happy about are:

1. GNM pinpoints the exact cause of a disease so none of those wishy-washy causes modern medicine likes to blame. Your genes, your lifestyle, your genes, oh yeh did I mention your genes?

2. GNM takes the fear out of cancer to the point where people will refuse modern medicine's disgusting, degrading and mutilating treatments taking their custom elsewhere. Goodbye profit margin.

For just these two reasons he had to be stopped. He was chased out of his country and even imprisoned for a time for trying to help people who had already been through conventional treatments or some who never would submit to them anyway. No money lost for them then. So far Dr Hamer just seemed to be mopping up the cancer industry's mess instead of leaving it under the rug where they wanted it.

Fast forward to 2022 and where is GNM now?

But first I'm sure you'd like to know what all the fuss is about. So here's a brief and simplified explanation of GNM 'dogma' sorry, yes sarcasm is the lowest form of wit.

GNM in one paragraph.

We all know what 'instinct' is don't we? Well GNM is a kind of instinct in the physical body. It's a survival mechanism we all have programmed in us, animals too, to deal with threats. Originally they were probably only physical threats but with our modern lives those physical threats may be attached to our home, family and other day to day issues.

This program kicks in instinctively to bolster our chances of surviving said threat. But only if we are genuinely caught off guard and resolving the threat is beyond our control. It may build tissue up in a region or it may dismantle tissue in another for a short term boost of physical power/strength to get us out of danger. Once the threat is resolved the process reverses.

This process produces a mark on the brain which can be seen on a CT scan and which shows where in the body the process is working and how far along the process it is.

The two phases can make themselves felt (symptoms) depending on the organ and what the particular process entails at which point modern medicine will tell you, you have a deadly disease with a fancy Latin name, an *itis or simply cancer, and so the nightmare begins…

Obviously that is very simplified, just so you know the kernel of what it's about and for time's sake I've barely scratched the surface.

There has been much coming and going in GNM from its beginning to now. Some people jumped in took what they could get then jumped out again and went off on their own path. Some even took to expanding Hamer's work with their own ideas based on nothing but the will to succeed, not necessarily in curing anyone, just succeeding. GNM is not a cure. It is a process that has always been there, just misunderstood until now. Anyone who claims it is a cure-all is selling you lies.

If you google GNM you will see the same faces splattered all over YouTube. Ask yourself why YouTube allows these people to openly tout their versions of GNM when the creator of it got put in a very real prison as opposed to a virtual one and the true GNM teachers can't even get their website listed on Google. Some are even doing consultations for money, selling books and teaching their own versions of GNM without having any qualifications to do so. Would you go to a self-taught doctor?

Most of these YT GNM 'doctors' seemed to magically pop up straight after the untimely death of Dr Hamer. Some are even weaving in their own dietary advise with it (GNM does not advise specific diets at all).

Just as I would never give medical advice on here you should not take any advice without checking their records first.

On all search engines the first website that comes up is one called 'Learning GNM'. It all looks very official and has lots of pages on specific 'symptoms and diagnosis' but again, buyer beware. It is I'm told NOT accurate. Not wrong enough to alert a newbie but wrong enough to cause possible harm yes.

Up until now there have been few alternatives where Joe Public can go to try and make sense of their own sickness. I too went to 'Learning GNM' and thought it helped me. But when things didn't seem to change I realised it hadn't helped. I needed someone who could really get to the bottom of my case. At which point I found the official GNM people. On the official GNM learning website there is an intro to GNM, a bit longer and more accurate than mine. [137]

---

[137] www.newmedicine.ca/german-new-medicine.php

It doesn't seem to come up on web searches. Funny that.

Even less funny is the old 'this site is not secure' warning. I remember that old ruse. It was used extensively on alternative truth, medicine and anti-vaccine sites to scare off the uninitiated. I used to look at it as a badge of honour back then. It obviously still is.

🔖   ⚠ Not secure | newmedicine.ca/statement2.php

These charlatans hogging the top search engine result pages must be being left alone because they are harming the future of GNM. They may not know they are harming it and there's the rub – are they controlled opposition if they don't know they are? People like me and many others who think they are learning the basics may be learning lies and sadly some are even being charged for it too. That's when it becomes not just negligent but fraudulent. A scam. Where did these people learn GNM? From the same website – 'Learning GNM.

Here is GNM's official say on Markolin and why she is not recommended and nor are her many self-taught 'students': [138]

> Caroline Markolin claims to be the GNM "authority" equal to Dr. Hamer. Dr. Hamer has never given her any kind of authority. Caroline Markolin, according to Dr. Hamer and his seminar attendance records, has taken two weeks of seminar with him and yet she presents a "certificate of attendance" as proof of her GNM knowledge and teaching expertise as if it gave her the permission from Dr. Hamer to exclusively give lectures and seminars in the English speaking world.
>
> Caroline Markolin does not have the body of knowledge or as Dr. Hamer says "a single day of clinical experience" to be able to call herself an expert in the GNM. It is for that reason that we at this website, which was originally established in 2001 by request of Dr. Hamer, have been asked to make this statement. Dr. Hamer recently mentioned to Ilsedora Laker that Caroline Markolin led him to believe that she was a PhD of biology when in fact her subject is German Literature. She does not have an official science background.

If GNM is to succeed we need to spread it by word of mouth just like the charlatans are but we need to point them to the real GNM. We need to do what they are doing, reach out on social media and we need the official people to come out from their GNM schools and meet the public, talk about GNM in simple terms. Do podcasts and interviews (yes coming soon). We don't need a sales pitch, GNM will sell itself because it is factual and it makes sense if it is not watered down or messed about with to fit someone's agenda. But we need to see the real deal and have them meet us on our own social media grounds. We can't shut up the charlatans because GNM is not regulated like modern

---

[138] Excerpt from: www.newmedicine.ca/statement2.php
Full statement here: www.newmedicine.ca/statement2.php

medicine (yet) but we can learn from their success by copying their promotion methods. Beat them at their own game so to speak.

Now that the cat is out of the bag I expect to see all the German videos on YouTube translated into English and Ilsedora Laker getting her face out there (or her trusted spokespersons at least) to let people know where they can go to get some real help until we have a GNM certified practitioner in every town. So far we have exactly zero in Ireland.

I like Lanka's idea of letting it grow organically alongside the other modalities as he says it sells itself, people will see what works and naturally move towards it. I especially liked his idea of a brain scanner without radiation and hopefully without having to go through modern medicine to get one.

I do believe we are at a crossroads now in health care and 'sickness' management. The crossroads also means we can go backwards. We don't want to do that and the only real way forwards is to take real GNM and the real Terrain theory with us.

No-one's saying this will be easy. It's up to you to fight for what you want especially when vested interests will fight you all the way. Onwards and upwards as they say. [139]

THE END

---

[139] www.gnmonlineseminars.com/

Thank you for buying this book. As we all know, important information can and does disappear from the internet but we'll always have books!

Please don't forget to leave a review if you enjoyed this one.

Printed in Great Britain
by Amazon